KT-222-581

WITHDRAWN

NAPIER UNIVERSITY LIS

Working with women and AIDS

MORNINGSIDE SITE LIBRARY
LOTHIAN COLLEGE OF HEALTH STUDIES
CANAAN LANE
EDINBURGH
EH10 4TB

'I welcome this book as a valuable account of the practical, policy and personal issues which have confronted women working with women, as the HIV epidemic has spread .... I am impressed and moved that several women who are HIV positive have had the courage to describe openly their feelings and personal needs. Their frank testimony, together with the authoritative commentary of so many of those who have pioneered special work on Women and HIV/AIDS, make this a powerful document in the chronicle of AIDS.'

Margaret Jay, writing in the Foreword

Women now account for one-third of the ten million people with HIV infection worldwide. On World AIDS Day in December 1990 the World Health Organisation estimated that three million women are currently HIV-infected and are expected to die by the year 2000. Yet until recently women have found that the available information often did not apply to them, that most services were geared towards men and that doctors and other professionals were often unprepared for the particular issues that women would raise.

Working with Women and AIDS fills this important gap by providing factual information and practical advice about medical, social and counselling issues concerning women and HIV infection. It explores questions of relevance to those working with women affected by HIV and AIDS: Are women more likely to be infected heterosexually than men? What are the implications for childbearing? What has the impact of AIDS been on women working in the sex industry? Do women with HIV infection have different emotional needs from men?

Written by people working in the field as well as by women who are themselves HIV positive, *Working with Women and AIDS* provides a unique and readable combination of up-to-date medical information, a discussion of social issues, personal accounts and practical suggestions about ways of working with women affected by HIV and AIDS. It will be invaluable to a wide range of health care professionals including counsellors, social workers, doctors and nurses, and will also be of great interest to lecturers and students in social policy as well as in the health care field.

Judy Bury is the Primary Care Facilitator (HIV/AIDS) for the Lothian Health Board; **Val Morrison** is a Research Psychologist in Health Psychology at the University of St Andrews; and **Sheena McLachlan** is a Project Worker with the Women and HIV/AIDS Network in Lothian.

Working with women and AIDS

Medical, social, and counselling issues

Edited by Judy Bury, Val Morrison and
Sheena McLachlan

Foreword by Margaret Jay

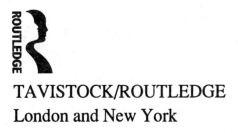

TAVISTOCK/ROUTLEDGE
London and New York

CA 362.19697920082 BUR

First published in 1992
by Routledge
11 New Fetter Lane, London EC4P 4EE

Simultaneously published in the USA and Canada
by Routledge
a division of Routledge, Chapman and Hall, Inc.
29 West 35th Street, New York, NY 10001

© 1992 Judy Bury, Val Morrison, Sheena McLachlan, the collection as
    a whole; each contributor, their chapter.
© Foreword 1992 Maragaret Jay

Typeset in 10/12pt Times by Michael Mepham, Frome, Somerset
Printed and bound in Great Britain by
Biddles Ltd, Guildford and King's Lynn.

All rights reserved. No part of this book may be reprinted or reproduced
or utilized in any form or by any electronic, mechanical, or other means,
now known or hereafter invented, including photocopying and
recording, or in any information storage or retrieval system, without
permission in writing from the publishers.

British Library Cataloguing in Publication Data
A catalogue record for this book is available from the British Library.

Library of Congress Cataloging in Publication Data
Working with women and AIDS : medical, social, and counselling
    issues / edited by Judy Bury, Val Morrison, Sheena McLachlan;
    foreword by Margaret Jay
    p.   cm.
    Includes bibliographical references and index.
    1. AIDS (Disease)—Social aspects. 2. Women—Diseases.
    3. Women's health services. I. Bury, Judith. II. Morrison, Val,
    1961– . III. McLachlan, Sheena, 1951–
    RA644.A25W66   1992
    362.1'969792'0082—dc20   92–9967
                                                                CIP

ISBN 0–415–07658–7
        0–415–07659–5 (pbk)

Women still constitute the large bulk of the country's educators and care-givers, through roles of teachers, nurses, social workers, counsellors, girlfriends, wives and mothers. All persons in these positions shoulder a great responsibility. They are expected to overcome their own fears, become comfortable with sexual, drug and lifestyle issues, acquire wisdom, nurture and teach the young, comfort the fearful, and care for the sick. It's a tall order.

(C. Wofsy (1987) *Children with HIV and their Families: Report of Surgeon General's Workshop*, USA: US Department of Health and Human Services)

Contents

Tables and figures

Contributors

Joy Barlow (Roulston): Projects Manager for the Aberlour Child Care Trust in Scotland. Responsible for the development and management of two short-term residential recovery units for female substance misusers with their children. Has worked on issues of HIV/AIDS with women since 1985. Member of the Home Office Advisory Council on the Misuse of Drugs.

Kate Bisset: Studied medicine at Aberdeen University 1970–6. Following general practice training, specialised in community psychiatry for five years at Dingleton Hospital in the Scottish Borders. From 1986–91 was team leader with the City Hospital HIV Counselling Clinic, Edinburgh.

Judy Bury: Has worked in family planning, venereology, sexual counselling and general practice. Now working in a community drug service, offering HIV counselling, testing and monitoring to drug users. Also employed by Lothian Health Board to teach general practitioners about AIDS and drugs. Author of *Teenage Pregnancy in Britain*, Birth Control Trust, 1984. Member of Conference Group of Women and HIV/AIDS Network.

Ruth Gilfillan: Husband died in accident in February 1987 after nine years of marriage. They had used drugs socially and injected once or twice but they knew nothing about HIV or AIDS. She found out that she was infected with HIV a few days after his death. She has three children aged 12, 10 and 5 years.

Jennifer Gray: Trained marriage counsellor and worked from 1985–9 as nurse counsellor in the counselling clinic at City Hospital and Leith Hospital, Edinburgh. Involved in training counsellors in HIV/AIDS counselling skills and as facilitator for 'Buddies' support group for Scottish AIDS Monitor. Currently working as student counsellor at University of Edinburgh.

Mary Hepburn: Senior Lecturer in Women's Reproductive Health jointly in Departments of Obstetrics and Gynaecology/Social Policy and Social

Work, Glasgow University; Consultant Obstetrician and Gynaecologist, Glasgow Royal Maternity Hospital, in charge of service providing reproductive health care for women with severe social problems including drug use and for women infected or affected by HIV.

Netta Maciver: Formerly Principal Officer (Addiction and AIDS Services) with Strathclyde Social Work Department 1986–90. Previously worked in child abuse unit of Royal Scottish Society for the Prevention of Cruelty to Children (RSSPCC) and then Assistant Director of Social Work (residential and day care services) for Western Isles Island Council. Currently living in Madrid but continues to undertake consultancy work in the UK.

Sheena McLachlan: Project worker with Women and HIV/AIDS Network in Lothian and freelance trainer in communication skills. Previously HIV/AIDS Educator with Lothian Region Community Education Service. Involved in setting up the first community-based women's health self-help group in Edinburgh.

Ruth Morgan Thomas: Formerly Research Associate working on HIV/AIDS-related risks in the sex industry in Edinburgh with the Alcohol Research Group, University of Edinburgh. Currently Project Co-ordinator for Scot-PEP (Scottish Prostitutes Education Project), a peer-led education group engaged in health promotion through outreach and a drop-in centre for male and female prostitutes and those involved in the commercial sex industry.

Val Morrison: Graduated in Psychology in 1983. Ran centre for homeless substance abusers in Cambridge 1983–5. Research Associate with the Alcohol Research Group, University of Edinburgh 1985–91, studying the impact of HIV on changing patterns of illicit drug use in Edinburgh. Now research psychologist working in health psychology looking at coping with chronic disease. Member of Women and HIV/AIDS Network.

Edith Springer: Social worker and AIDS and drugs trainer in New York and New Jersey. Originally in the field of drug treatment, she left in the mid-1980s to concentrate on AIDS. Formerly supervised AIDS training of drug workers and is currently designing and performing psychosocial AIDS training for medical personnel. Also involved in several AIDS outreach projects focusing on homeless individuals in high drug use areas in New York City.

Kate Thomson: Project Manager at Positively Women since 1989. Previously much of her adult life was spent travelling and working abroad. Since returning to England in 1986 she has worked as a Support Worker for people with learning difficulties and most recently studied Communication Studies and Sociology at Goldsmiths College.

Jane Wilson: Senior clinical psychologist in Muirhouse/Pilton Drug Project, Edinburgh, working in the community with drug users who are infected or affected by HIV, their families and friends. Previously spent six years in San Francisco training in and working with both drug users and issues around HIV/AIDS. This included two years working in a women's polydrug abuse programme.

Foreword

Margaret Jay

'Women and AIDS' – a special subject with special significance. Only recently have the particular concerns of women infected and affected by the HIV virus been acknowledged and openly discussed, and, in the UK, the Scottish Women and HIV/AIDS Network have led the way. I welcome this book as a valuable account of the practical, policy and personal issues which have confronted women working with women, as the HIV epidemic has spread.

The book concentrates on the social and counselling issues which are of great importance to women. HIV is an alarmingly stigmatising virus and affected women often feel a special isolation and sense of social prejudice which adds almost intolerable burdens to already difficult lives. Women with children are specially vulnerable. It's difficult to persuade mothers to seek appropriate care and counselling for themselves in the face of genuine fears about the impact on their children. Often this has led to women seeking help and treatment only when their HIV disease is well advanced. We must all go on working to break down the attitudes which still make it impossible for women to come forward for help and support when they need it.

The recently published figures on anonymous screening for HIV in ante-natal clinics show how rapidly the numbers of infected pregnant women are growing. This presents an urgent problem of care for mothers and children in many different places in the UK, and the extensive Scottish experience, described in this book, must provide a framework of good practice to be followed everywhere.

However excellent the care and support for women with HIV-related illness, there is little immediate prospect of a cure or anti-viral vaccine; the only way to prevent further spread is through education and information. Educating young women to negotiate safer sex with their partners requires complex skills and an understanding far beyond the transmission of simple facts. The immediate need to expand this difficult work is, again, demonstrated by recent statistics which show that 40 per cent of AIDS cases among women in the UK are in the 15–29 age group, which means that most of them were infected in their teens, and yet young women in this age group seem to be the ones most resistant to adopting safer sex. In this field, as well as in care, the psychologists, doctors, counsellors and educators writing in this book contribute a wealth of experience to a vitally important subject.

Finally, I am impressed and moved that several women who are HIV positive have had the courage to describe openly their feelings and personal needs. Their frank testimony, together with the authoritative commentary of so many of those who have pioneered special work on Women and HIV/AIDS, make this a powerful document in the chronicle of AIDS.

Acknowledgements

The editors wish to thank their colleagues in the Women and HIV/AIDS Network who trusted them to edit this book on behalf of the Network. They are also indebted to Hazel Dawson, the Network administrator, for her word-processing skills, her patience and her support.

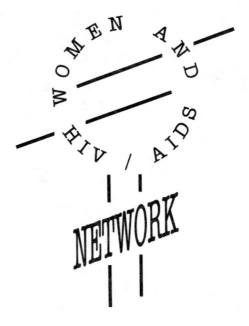

Introduction

This book arises out of four conferences held in Scotland between 1988 and 1991, organised by the Scottish Women and HIV/AIDS Network. The Network was established in 1988 with the aim of bringing together those working in the field of AIDS who were concerned about women's issues.

When AIDS was first described in the early 1980s, it was thought to be a disease that affected only gay men. It was not long before AIDS was recognised to be the same as the disease that was killing many people in Africa, both men and women. By 1982 it was accepted that AIDS had an infective cause and in 1984 the virus that was subsequently named HIV was isolated. Yet many people in the West continued to see AIDS as a disease of gay men, and assumed that other people, including women, would not be at risk – that somehow, inexplicably, Africa was different. Women were affected by AIDS, as friends, sisters, mothers, carers and sometimes as lovers of men with AIDS, but it was thought unlikely that women in the West would develop AIDS.

By 1985, it was clear that people in the West other than gay men were developing AIDS – people who had become infected through blood transfusions, needle-sharing drug users, babies of infected drug users and even people who had become infected through heterosexual intercourse. Women, heterosexual men and children were developing AIDS, and the fact that women were at risk could no longer be ignored. But as women became infected and began to look for information and support, they found that the information available often did not apply to them, that most services were geared towards men, and that doctors and other professionals were often unprepared for the particular issues that women would raise.

By the end of 1987 there were 371 women in Scotland who had tested positive for HIV. By the same date there were 779 women in the whole of the UK known to be HIV positive. Thus at that time women in Scotland accounted for almost half of all women in the UK who were known to have HIV infection. In January 1988 a group of women working in the AIDS field in Edinburgh decided to form a network to share knowledge about the implications of HIV and AIDS for women, and to share experience about working with women affected by HIV and AIDS. Since then, the Women and HIV/AIDS Network has grown to include people professionally or personally affected by AIDS from many parts of Scotland. The Network meets as a regular women-only forum, distributes a newsletter and organises seminars in local areas in order to disseminate information about the risk of HIV infection for women and the implications of HIV infection for women who are already infected. In addition, the Network organises annual national conferences which have attracted delegates from most parts of the UK and have brought together men and women working in the field and those infected or personally affected by HIV and AIDS.

The first conference was held in May 1988. Entitled 'Women and AIDS: Issues, Needs, Awareness', it addressed the implications of AIDS for women by presenting an overview of medical, social and counselling issues. At the second conference in 1989, more emphasis was placed on sharing knowledge and experience. The third conference in 1990 coincided with World AIDS Day which focused on Women and AIDS. This conference was residential, to encourage contact between delegates. The focus was more international and there was a greater contribution from women with HIV infection. In 1991 the Network organised a conference on medical aspects of women and HIV infection with the intention of raising awareness amongst medical professionals.

In the early days of the Network, there were those who asked why we were looking particularly at women's needs. They argued that 'AIDS is AIDS' regardless of whether it was affecting a man or a woman. Of course, the most obvious response to this is that women bear children and men do not. Once it became clear that women were at risk from AIDS, one of the first questions that was asked was about the implications of AIDS for childbearing. This important topic, where the information given to women has often been misleading or worse, is covered thoroughly in this book. But the ability to bear children is not the only factor that distinguishes women from men and, as the epidemic has progressed, it has become clear that there are many other questions to which women have wanted answers. Are women more likely to be infected heterosexually than men, and if so, why? Do HIV disease and AIDS follow a different course in women compared to men? What are the social factors that impinge on women infected or affected by HIV and AIDS? How have women in the sex industry been affected by this sexually trans-mitted infection? Do women with HIV infection have different emotional needs from men? What particular issues arise in counselling women? Do women as carers have to face different issues from men? These are just some of the topics that the Network has addressed and that are covered in this book.

This book does not attempt to provide a comprehensive picture of all issues relating to women and AIDS. For example, although the risk of an infected woman giving birth to an infected child is discussed in Chapter 4, the subject of children with HIV and AIDS is deserving of a book in its own right and hence is not discussed fully within this volume. In addition, although issues about AIDS for women from ethnic minorities and for lesbians are mentioned, they are not dealt with in depth. The book does, however, cover a wide range of topics which should be of interest and value to counsellors, social workers, drug workers, community workers, nurses, doctors, other health professionals and to students in all these fields. As HIV infection continues to spread throughout the community, people working in these fields in all parts of the country will be increasingly affected by the impact of this virus on their work and on their personal lives. Our contributors are women working directly with women affected by HIV and AIDS, and they come from a range of backgrounds including nursing, clinical psychology, social work, psychiatry, general practice, obstetrics, research, community education and counselling.

We are grateful to Margaret Jay, Director of the National AIDS Trust, for providing a Foreword. The Trust gave a generous grant to the Network during its early years and Margaret came to Edinburgh to open our second conference in 1989. She has been actively involved in campaigning and in directing AIDS-related work for many years and was one of the first people outside Scotland to acknowledge women's special needs.

The first part of the book sets the scene by examining some background issues concerning women and HIV/AIDS. In Chapter 1 Judy Bury provides a comprehensive picture of the extent of HIV infection amongst women both nationally and internationally and describes how this picture is likely to change as HIV continues to spread heterosexually. She also discusses the ways in which HIV infection manifests itself in women. In the second chapter Joy Barlow provides an overview of the social consequences of HIV infection and places some of these costs in the context of women's role in society. Edith Springer then broadens this picture in Chapter 3 in her consideration of the impact of HIV and AIDS on women in the United States, and in New York City in particular, where AIDS is now a major cause of death in women.

The second part of the book deals with the subjects of contraception and pregnancy. In Chapter 4 Judy Bury clarifies some of the important questions that are frequently asked about pregnancy, heterosexual transmission and contraception. Is pregnancy dangerous for infected women? What is the risk of a woman with HIV infection transmitting the infection to her baby? How is HIV infection transmitted sexually? What methods of contraception are suitable for women with HIV infection? In Chapter 5 Mary Hepburn outlines some of the ways in which women can be supported in making decisions about HIV testing, about drug use, about termination or about prospects for their child.

The third section discusses prostitution or sex work. In the early days of the epidemic, the only interest directed at prostitutes was in order to blame them for the spread of HIV infection. In the sixth chapter Ruth Morgan Thomas provides an overview of the nature of sex work and discusses society's perceptions of the sex industry. She demonstrates that, rather than blaming sex workers for the spread of HIV infection, it is important to recognise that they are more at risk of being infected by HIV than of infecting others and, in addition, that sex workers can be an important resource for HIV prevention. In Chapter 7 Netta Maciver describes the response that one city has made to the needs of prostitutes, and provides practical guidelines and suggestions about how to set up a facility which attracts women and enables them to protect themselves and their clients from infection.

The fourth section of the book concentrates on the issues that need to be considered when planning educational strategies or providing counselling. In Chapter 8 Judy Bury discusses the psychosocial issues that make it difficult for women to protect themselves against HIV infection. She goes on to look at the implications of these issues for sex education and for mass media campaigns. These issues are taken further by Jane Wilson in Chapter 9 where she considers what must be taken into account when counselling women, especially women from drug-using communities, about safer sex. She includes a detailed analysis of the factors that discourage women from coming for counselling as well as those factors that interfere with effective work once women are in counselling. In considering counselling it is essential to acknowledge the needs of counsellors themselves. In Chapter 10, Jane Wilson discusses the needs of women as carers, and explores why we find it so difficult to have these needs met.

The final section of the book is concerned with the feelings and needs of women with HIV infection and AIDS. In Chapter 11 Kate Bisset and Jennifer Gray describe the emotions that may be experienced by women before and after an HIV antibody test and some of the responses – shock, denial, isolation, hurt, anger, depression – that women may have to a positive diagnosis. They also emphasise the importance of support. Kate Thomson in Chapter 12 describes how her own diagnosis led her to become involved in setting up Positively Women, an organisation run by women for women who are HIV positive or have AIDS. The book ends with the poetry of Ruth Gilfillan where we are reminded of the vulnerability of infected women, the isolation, the guilt and anxieties, the anger, the fears, and yet strength that can permeate a woman's life and relationships.

One question that might be asked by a potential reader of this book is 'Why Scotland?' What relevance does the Scottish experience have to the rest of the United Kingdom, let alone anywhere else? There are certainly some ways in which our experience in Scotland is very different from other areas. For example, women from ethnic minorities are under-represented and the vast majority of infected women in Scotland are white. Scotland, and Edinburgh in particular, has a disproportionate number of women with HIV infection. Edinburgh, with 1 per cent of the female UK population accounts for 19 per cent of women known to be HIV infected. As a result, there have been developments in the care of women, and painful lessons have been learned, that will be of relevance to many other areas. Recent evidence from anonymous antenatal screening (see Chapter 4) suggests that there are other areas of the country where women are becoming infected in large numbers and in certain parts of London the prevalence of HIV infection among women is now as high as in Edinburgh (Medical Research Council, 1991). We need to remain alert. We need to learn from each other. This book goes some way towards sharing what we have already learned.

    Judy Bury   *Sheena McLachlan*   *Val Morrison*

REFERENCE

Medical Research Council (1991) 'The unlinked anonymous HIV prevalence monitoring programme in England and Wales; preliminary results', *Communicable Disease Report* 1: 69–76.

Part I
Background issues

1 Women and the AIDS epidemic
Some medical facts and figures

Judy Bury

Today, the proportion of women affected worldwide is growing fast, but awareness about the ways in which HIV affects women and the services they need lags behind.

(Panos Institute 1990)

On World AIDS Day in December 1990 the World Health Organisation estimated that 'three million women are currently HIV infected and are expected to die by the year 2000' (World Health Organisation 1990). AIDS has become the leading cause of death for women aged 20–40 in major cities in Western Europe, in the Americas and in sub-Saharan Africa.

In this chapter I shall consider the extent of HIV infection amongst women in the United Kingdom, and how this picture is likely to change over the next few years as HIV infection continues to spread heterosexually. The situation for women in the UK will be considered in relation to the effects of HIV and AIDS on women worldwide. I shall then go on to discuss the physical effects of HIV and AIDS on women, and factors that affect the survival of women with AIDS. Finally I shall discuss the official classification of AIDS and research into AIDS (including trials of new drugs), both areas in which women suffer discrimination.

WOMEN, AIDS AND HIV INFECTION IN THE UK

In the UK up to the end of 1991 only 5 per cent of adults who had developed AIDS were women. From Table 1.1 it can be seen that the vast majority of people with AIDS in the UK are gay men. Together with haemophiliacs (almost all men), they account for 84 per cent of people with AIDS. Even among drug users with AIDS, men outnumber women by almost three to one.

In Scotland, women account for 12 per cent of adults with AIDS. From Table 1.2 it can be seen that gay men and haemophiliacs account for only 54 per cent of those with AIDS in Scotland. Compared to the UK as a whole,

Table 1.1 Adult AIDS cases in UK up to 31.12.91

How persons probably acquired the virus	Male	Female	
Sexual intercourse between men	4,197	–	
Injecting drug use (IDU)	176	69	
IDU and sexual intercourse between men	83	–	
Haemophiliac	286	4	
Blood products	30	46	
Heterosexual contact abroad	228	116	
Heterosexual contact in the UK	49	49	
Other/undetermined	61	8	
Total	5,110	292	(5%)

Source: Adapted from *Answer* (AIDS News Supplement, CDS Weekly Report) CDS 92/04

a much higher proportion of those with AIDS in Scotland have acquired the infection by sharing injecting equipment or through unprotected heterosexual intercourse (41 per cent compared to 13 per cent).

On average it takes ten years from becoming infected with HIV to the development of AIDS (Rutherford *et al.* 1990). Thus, looking at those who have AIDS now tells us about who was becoming infected ten years ago. To know more about who is becoming infected with HIV now, we need to look at those known to be HIV positive, which in turn will tell us something about the nature of the AIDS epidemic in approximately ten years from now.

Although women account for only 5 per cent of the AIDS cases in the UK, they account for 12 per cent of those currently known to be HIV positive (CDSC 1992). It is striking that in the UK gay men and haemophiliacs account for 68 per cent of those known to have HIV infection compared to 84 per cent of those with AIDS, and those who have become infected through sharing needles or through heterosexual intercourse account for 24 per cent of those known to have HIV infection compared to 13 per cent of those with AIDS. Thus as the epidemic progresses women will represent an increasing

Table 1.2 Adult AIDS cases in Scotland up to 31.12.91

How persons probably acquired the virus	Male	Female	
Sexual intercourse between men	136	–	
Injecting drug use (IDU)	66	25	
Haemophiliac	16	–	
Blood products	5	3	
Heterosexual contact abroad	15	1	
Heterosexual contact in the UK	4	5	
Other/undetermined	4	–	
Total	246	34	(12%)

Source: Adapted from *Answer* (AIDS News Supplement, CDS Weekly Report) CDS 92/04

proportion of those with AIDS and by the turn of the century more than one in ten of those developing AIDS in the UK will be women.

In Scotland women account for 12 per cent of adults with AIDS but for 27 per cent of those known to be HIV positive. Gay men and haemophiliacs account for 24 per cent of those known to have HIV infection compared to 54 per cent of those with AIDS. People who have become infected through sharing needles or through heterosexual intercourse account for 63 per cent of those known to be HIV positive compared to 41 per cent of those with AIDS. The indications are that by the turn of the century more than a quarter of those developing AIDS in Scotland will be women. The differences between Scotland and the UK as a whole are summarised in Table 1.3.

Table 1.3 Scotland and the United Kingdom – a comparison

| | UK | | Scotland | |
	AIDS	HIV	AIDS	HIV
Gay men and haemophiliacs	84%	68%	54%	24%
Needle sharing/heterosexual intercourse	13%	24%	41%	63%
Women as % of total cases	5%	12%	12%	27%

The AIDS epidemic in Europe and the United States has come in waves. The first wave of the epidemic was gay men. The second wave was injecting drug users where HIV infected men outnumbered women by three to one. Looking again at people with AIDS in Scotland (Table 1.2) we can see that there are more gay men than injecting drug users. But if we look at those known to be HIV positive in Scotland (Table 1.4), it is clear that injecting drug users will soon outnumber gay men among the cases of AIDS. The third

Table 1.4 HIV-antibody positive reports in Scotland up to 31.12.91

How persons probably acquired the virus	Male	Female
Sexual intercourse between men	365	–
Injecting drug use (IDU)	661	305
IDU and sexual intercourse between men	7	–
Haemophiliac	78	–
Blood products	6	7
Heterosexual contact abroad	26	12
Heterosexual contact in the UK	56	106
Other/undetermined	159	69
Total	1,358	499 (27%)

Source: Adapted from *Answer* (AIDS News Supplement, CDS Weekly Report) CDS 92/04

wave of the epidemic will be AIDS cases resulting from heterosexual transmission which, as we shall see, will involve women more than men.

WOMEN, DRUG USE AND HIV IN SCOTLAND

In the early 1980s Scotland seemed to be escaping the worst of the AIDS epidemic. There were some gay men with AIDS, particularly in the larger cities, Glasgow and Edinburgh. Many of these men had become infected elsewhere and there did not seem to be any large-scale indigenous sexual spread. Then, between 1983 and 1985, a particular combination of circumstances in Edinburgh – a rapid increase in the number of young people injecting drugs for the first time, the unavailability of needles and syringes, and the popularity of shooting galleries – meant that, when HIV infection entered the drug-using community, it spread rapidly (Robertson *et al.* 1986). By 1985 50 per cent of injecting drug users had become infected, one-third of them women (Robertson *et al.* 1986). By 1987, not only did Edinburgh have 30 per cent of all women in the UK known to be infected with HIV, but Edinburgh also had the highest prevalence of HIV infection of anywhere in the UK (Lothian Health Board 1988). In Glasgow, the availability of injecting equipment has often been cited as the reason for the lower levels of seroprevalence among drug users (e.g. Green *et al.* 1991), but concern remains that these levels could suddenly increase if needle-sharing practices were to change. Recent research has shown a decrease in the sharing of injecting equipment in Edinburgh (e.g. Robertson *et al.* 1988, Morrison 1991) but there has not been a parallel change in sexual behaviour (Morrison 1991).

WOMEN AND HETEROSEXUAL TRANSMISSION

In the UK as a whole the number of people infected heterosexually increased by 20 per cent between December 1989 and December 1990. Of all adults newly identified as having HIV infection in 1990, 19 per cent were infected heterosexually. In Edinburgh in 1990 and 1991 more people became infected with HIV through heterosexual transmission than by any other means. It seems that gay men have changed their behaviour and drug users are less likely to inject or share needles than they were but there has not yet been a significant change in heterosexual behaviour. Thus it is likely that heterosexual spread will continue for the next few years at least.

Many people continue to ignore the reality of heterosexual transmission. This complacency was seriously challenged by the publication in 1991 of the results of anonymous HIV testing of pregnant women which revealed that in some parts of London as many as one woman in two hundred is now infected with HIV (Medical Research Council 1991).

What is the significance of heterosexual transmission for women? Whether we look at the UK figures or at the Scottish figures, it is clear that more women are becoming infected heterosexually within the UK than men, by a ratio of nearly two to one. More than two-thirds of these positive reports have been since 1987. This is the third wave of the epidemic.

As more people are becoming infected heterosexually and as more women are becoming infected heterosexually than men, the proportion of those with HIV infection who are women is increasing and will continue to increase.

Why are women more likely to be infected by heterosexual transmission than men? One reason is that an infected man is slightly more likely to infect a woman during sexual intercourse than the other way around (Johnson 1990) but a more important reason is that at present more heterosexual men are infected than women so that women are far more likely to encounter an infected man than vice versa. If we take Edinburgh as an example, it has been estimated that 1 in 100 men aged 15 to 45 years is now infected with HIV compared to 1 in 250 women (Lothian Health Board 1989). Thus a woman in Edinburgh is more than twice as likely to meet an infected man than a man is to meet an infected woman.

Since we are relatively near the beginning of the heterosexual epidemic in the UK, it is still the case that the majority of women with HIV infection are injecting drug users or their partners. As heterosexual spread continues, this pattern will change but currently most women with HIV infection are, like the majority of injecting drug users, from areas of deprivation. Injecting drug use is in part a reflection of 'frustration and anger of marginalized and impoverished populations seeking escape through mood-altering drugs' (Panos Institute 1990). In Scotland, most multiply-deprived people are White and in many parts of the UK deprivation is not linked with race. In the US however deprivation is more closely associated with race. As in the UK, the majority of women with AIDS are injecting drug users or their partners and nearly three-quarters of women with AIDS are Black or Hispanic compared to less than half of men. Thus, in the US, as in the UK, AIDS and drug use are associated with deprivation which has added implications for women who are infected. These are discussed in Chapters 2 and 3.

WOMEN AND HIV INFECTION – THE GLOBAL PICTURE

It is important to see the situation for women in the UK in relation to the epidemic worldwide. Globally, it is estimated that approximately one-third of all those with HIV infection are women. It has been predicted however

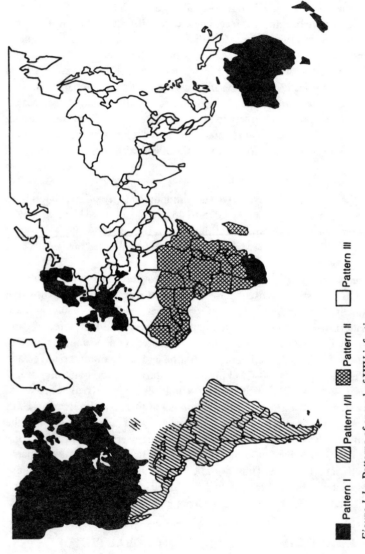

Figure 1.1 Patterns of spread of HIV infection
Source: Sato *et al.* 1989

■ Pattern I ▨ Pattern I/II ▨ Pattern II ☐ Pattern III

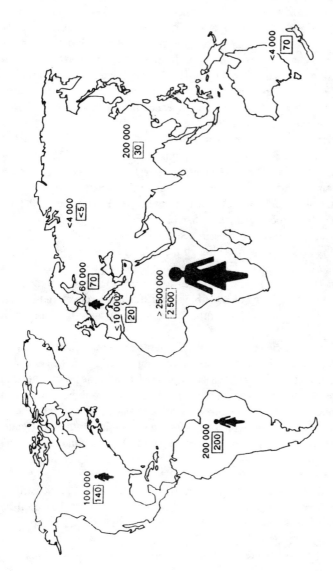

Figure 1.2 Estimated number of HIV-infected women aged 15–49 years. No. in boxes = prevalence per 100,000 women
Source: World Health Organisation 1991

that by the year 2000 there will be nearly as many women with AIDS as men (World Health Organisation 1990).

During the mid-1980s the World Health Organisation (WHO) identified regions of the world according to the predominant mode of HIV spread. The pattern of spread of HIV infection in the UK and North America is similar to that seen in the whole of Western Europe and in Australia and New Zealand. In all these areas, extensive spread of HIV infection began in the late 1970s and early 1980s and most of those infected up to now have been homosexual men or injecting drug users. Although heterosexual spread is increasing it still accounts for relatively few infections. It has been estimated that more than 100,000 women in these countries, known as pattern I countries, are infected (Chin 1990).

In sub-Saharan Africa, known as pattern II countries, extensive spread of HIV infection probably began in the mid- to late 1970s and is found predominantly in sexually active heterosexuals. In these countries there are as many women with AIDS as men and it has been estimated that more than two million women, mostly of childbearing age, have been infected with HIV (Chin 1990). It has been estimated that 10 per cent of those with AIDS in sub-Saharan Africa have become infected from transfusions with infected blood (Panos Institute 1990). Although the risks are now known and those most at risk of being infected are advised not to donate blood, it is still not possible in many developing countries to screen all blood. Women are disproportionately affected as most blood transfusions in developing countries are given to women for complications of pregnancy and childbirth (Panos Institute 1990).

Many Latin American and Caribbean countries were initially classified as pattern I but heterosexual transmission has increased to such an extent in these areas that they are now classified as pattern I/II. In some Latin American countries, a signficant number of men have intercourse with both sexes and in these countries more women have become infected through intercourse with bisexual men than through intercourse with injecting drug users (Panos Institute 1990). The proportion of women with HIV infection is increasing and it has been estimated that more than 200,000 women in Latin America are now infected (Chin 1990).

Pattern III countries are those where HIV was introduced in the early to mid-1980s, where prevalence has been low and where there has been no clearly predominant mode of spread. Such areas include Asia, Pacific countries other than Australia and New Zealand, Eastern Europe, North Africa and the Middle East. However, in some countries the situation is changing rapidly. For example, at the end of the 1980s, HIV infection spread rapidly among intravenous drug users in South East Asia, and among female prostitutes in several cities in Thailand and India. In Thailand the ratio of female to male HIV infection rose from one to seventeen in 1986 to one to five in 1990 (Panos Insitute 1990). In Bombay nearly one-quarter of women working in the sex industry are now infected (Panos Institute 1990). It has been estimated that there are nearly 300,000 women with HIV infection in these areas (Chin 1990).

The WHO classification provides only a broad picture of the epidemic as patterns of infection vary from one country to another within some regions. The classification has also required revision, and will probably require further revision, as patterns of infection change.

The impact of the epidemic on communities in different parts of the world may vary but the impact of HIV infection and AIDS on the individual woman is fundamentally the same.

THE PHYSICAL EFFECTS OF HIV INFECTION ON WOMEN

HIV infection mostly follows the same pattern in men and women. Between a few days and a few months after infection, around the time that the HIV antibody test becomes positive, there may be a short illness like flu or glandular fever (Leen and Brettle 1991). This 'seroconversion illness' is only experienced by a minority of those who become infected. People with HIV infection then remain well for some years before developing symptoms of HIV disease. Early symptoms include enlarged lymph nodes, weight loss, fevers, sweats and diarrhoea. This combination of symptoms is sometimes known as AIDS-Related Complex (ARC) although this term is being used less and less. As HIV infection continues to damage the immune system, the body is less able to defend itself against infections (known as opportunistic infections) and cancer. AIDS (Acquired Immune Deficiency Syndrome) is diagnosed once one of a number of conditions has developed which indicates severe immune damage, such as *Pneumocystis carinii* pneumonia (PCP) or Kaposi's sarcoma (KS). These conditions are defined by the Centers for Disease Control in Atlanta, Georgia in the US. Studies suggest that on average it takes ten years for someone with HIV infection to develop AIDS (e.g. Moss and Bacchetti 1989, Rutherford *et al.* 1990); that is, 50 per cent of people will develop AIDS within ten years of infection with HIV while 50 per cent of people with HIV infection will take longer than ten years to develop AIDS. In fact, these figures come from studies of HIV infection in gay men – similar research has not been done on drug users or women with HIV infection.

Women experience the same spectrum of illnesses associated with AIDS apart from Kaposi's sarcoma (KS). This slowly progressing skin cancer, which is a common manifestation of AIDS in men, seems to be a sexually transmitted condition (Beral *et al.* 1990) which is only rarely seen in those

LOTHIAN COLLEGE OF HEALTH STUDIES LIBRARY

who have acquired HIV infection through needle sharing (Leen and Brettle 1991). Women who have acquired HIV infection heterosexually are more likely to have KS if their partners are bisexual men than if they are injecting drug users (Beral *et al.* 1990) and women may also develop KS if they have become infected by a blood transfusion (Lassoued *et al.* 1991). Although uncommon in women, when it does develop it may spread more rapidly than in men and can be fatal (Lassoued *et al.* 1991).

People with HIV disease are particularly prone to infections with candida (thrush). In men or women this can affect the mouth or oesophagus (gullet) and in women it can also affect the vagina. Vaginal thrush (candidiasis) is very common in women with HIV infection (Rhoads *et al.* 1987). It often recurs after treatment and may become severe and unresponsive to treatment as HIV disease progresses (Brettle and Leen 1991).

Women with HIV infection are also more likely to develop other gynaecological infections. Genital warts, genital herpes and pelvic inflammatory disease are all common in women with HIV infection and, like thrush, they may be recurrent and severe (Brettle and Leen 1991). Once the immune system has been severely damaged, the body may not be able to respond to an infection in the normal way, by causing pain and inflammation, so that the diagnosis may be missed (ACT UP 1991). Continuing untreated infection may then cause further damage to the immune system (ACT UP 1991).

Women with HIV infection have been found to be more likely to develop abnormal cervical smears (cervical dysplasia) and possibly cervical cancer, apparently related to the increased incidence of genital herpes infection (Centers for Disease Control 1990). Continuing immune damage is associated with increasing abnormalities of cervical cells (Brettle and Leen 1991). It is interesting to note however that there has been no increase in the incidence of cervical cancer in New York and cervical cancer is rarely listed as a cause of HIV-related death. Nevertheless, it is advisable for women with HIV infection to be offered regular and frequent (at least annual) cervical smears.

Recurrent chest infections are common in HIV infected drug users, many of whom are women, and this is often the way in which severe HIV disease presents in women (Brettle and Leen 1991).

Some studies have found that women are more likely than men to experience severe weight loss associated with HIV disease (Brettle and Leen 1991). Both men and women may also experience thinning of the hair. These problems can cause particular emotional distress to women, who tend to be more concerned than men about their appearance.

The particular issues that relate to contraception, pregnancy and childbearing for women with HIV infection will be dealt with in Chapter 4.

SURVIVAL OF WOMEN WITH AIDS

A number of studies of survival of people with AIDS have found that women survive a significantly shorter time after a diagnosis of AIDS than men (e.g. Rothenberg *et al.* 1987) and Black women drug users survive the shortest time of all (Rothenberg *et al.* 1987). Over the last few years men and women have been living longer after a diagnosis of AIDS but in studies in the UK and the US women still survive for a shorter time than men (Lemp *et al.* 1990, Willocks *et al.* 1991).

Shorter survival in women could be due to a number of factors. AIDS sometimes takes a much slower course in men who present with Kaposi's sarcoma which is a rare presentation in women (see p. 17). Women tend to come forward later in the disease than men, particularly in the US where they have poorer access to health care due to poverty (see Chapter 3). Poor minority women in particular are unlikely to be receiving ongoing preventive medical care and may be reluctant to seek help when they are ill (ACT UP 1991). Women may also be slow to come forward because they consider their own health needs after the needs of their family. Doctors may contribute to the poor survival of women as they are sometimes slow to recognise symptoms of AIDS when they present in women and may give them inappropriate treatment. In addition, women are less likely to be offered new drug treatments (see p. 20). Another possible explanation for shorter survival could be biological differences between men and women in disease progression (ACT UP 1991).

A recent study in Edinburgh compared the progression of HIV infection in male and female drug users of similar background where all had been receiving good medical care. Even here male drug users were found to survive longer after a diagnosis of AIDS than female drug users (Willocks *et al.* 1991). The authors commented that since many of the women were principle carers for children they 'may receive less prophylactic and pre-AIDS care' (Willocks *et al.* 1991). There is clearly a need for more research into the natural history of HIV disease in women.

CLASSIFICATION OF AIDS AND WOMEN

As discussed previously, the diagnosis of AIDS depends on the appearance of one of a number of conditions that are defined by the Centers for Disease Control (CDC). Although this list of conditions was broadened in 1987, it still does not include any of the gynaecological conditions that are associated with HIV infection in women (see p. 18). Thus women may die from HIV-associated conditions without a diagnosis of AIDS. In a recent study of deaths of women with HIV/AIDS in the US it was found that 48 per cent died of conditions not listed in the CDC definition for AIDS (Chu 1990).

The exclusion of gynaecological conditions from the current definition of AIDS has a number of results. First, women are under-represented in AIDS statistics. Second, in countries such as the US where certain benefits are only available once someone has an AIDS diagnosis, many women with severe HIV disease will not be eligible for benefits. Third, many women with severe HIV disease are excluded from trials of new drugs, as some of these are only given to those with an AIDS diagnosis.

WOMEN, DRUG TRIALS AND RESEARCH

There are very few drugs that have been approved for the treatment of HIV disease and AIDS. Many new drugs are under trial and, for some people with HIV disease, the only access to drug treatment may be to take part in the trial of a new drug. Yet much research on new drugs for HIV disease is limited to men. Even women with an AIDS diagnosis are often excluded from drug trials for fear that they may become pregnant during the treatment and the drug might damage the foetus. They are only included in trials of some drugs if they are using 'adequate birth control' which sometimes requires sterilisation (ACT UP 1991).

Some drug trials do include women but the trial design rarely includes questions about the effect of the drug on menstruation, or on the progression of gynaecological conditions such as vaginal thrush, pelvic infection or cervical cancer (ACT UP 1991). Some women have noticed that drugs used for the treatment of AIDS such as AZT (Zidovudine) and ddI can cause painful, heavy and prolonged periods but these effects have not been studied (ACT UP 1991).

HIV/AIDS is still a relatively new disease and a great deal of research has been and is being conducted in order to understand more about the various manifestations of HIV infection and AIDS. Women are clearly under-represented in this research and although some researchers recognise that there is a lack of knowledge about the course of HIV infection and AIDS in women (e.g. Brettle and Leen 1991) women are still being excluded from much of the relevant research. This is increasingly inexcusable as women are increasingly affected by HIV and AIDS.

REFERENCES

ACT UP (1991) *Treatment and Research Agenda for Women with HIV Infection*, US: AIDS Coalition to Unleash Power.

Beral, V., Peterman, T.A., Berkelman, R.L. and Jaffe, H.W. (1990) 'Kaposi's sarcoma among persons with AIDS: a sexually transmitted infection?', *Lancet* 335: 123-8.

Brettle, R.P. and Leen, C.L.S. (1991) 'The natural history of HIV and AIDS in women', *AIDS* 5: 1283-92.

Centers for Disease Control (1990) 'Risk for cervical disease in HIV-infected women – New York City', *Morbidity and Mortality Weekly Report* 39(47): 846-9.

CDSC (1992) 'AIDS and HIV-1 infection: United Kingdom', *Communicable Disease Report* 2(4): 17-20.

Chin, J. (1990) 'Current and future dimensions of the HIV/AIDS pandemic in women and children', *Lancet* 336: 221-4.

Chu, S.Y., Buehler, J.W. and Berkelman, R.L. (1990) 'Impact of the human immunodeficiency virus epidemic on mortality in women of reproductive age, United States', *Journal of the American Medical Association* 264(2): 225-9.

Green, S.T., Willocks, L.J. and Leen, C.L.S. (1991) 'The appearance of HIV among Edinburgh and Glasgow injecting drug users: why do the HIV dissemination patterns differ so much between the two cities?', *Answer* (AIDS News Supplement, CDS Weekly Report) 91/09.

Johnson, A. (1990) 'The epidemiology of HIV in the UK: sexual transmission', in *HIV and AIDS: An Assessment of Current and Future Spread in the UK*, UK Health Departments and Health Education Authority, London: HMSO.

Lassoued, K., Clauvel, J.-P., Fegueux, S., Matheron, S., Gorin, I. and Oksenhendler, E. (1991) 'AIDS-associated Kaposi's sarcoma in female patients', *AIDS* 5: 877-80.

Leen, C.L.S. and Brettle, R.P. (1991) 'Natural history of HIV Infection', in G. Bird (ed.) *Imunology of HIV Infection*, London: Kluwer Press.

Lemp, G.F., Payne, S.F., Neal, D., Temelso, T. and Rutherford, G.W. (1990) 'Survival trends for patients with AIDS', *Journal of the American Medical Association* 263(3): 402-6.

Lothian Health Board (1988) *AIDS in Lothian: Everyone's Concern*, Edinburgh.

Lothian Health Board (1989) *AIDS in Lothian: Time to TAKE CARE*, Edinburgh.

Medical Research Council (1991) 'The unlinked anonymous HIV prevalence monitoring programme in England and Wales: preliminary results', *Communicable Disease Report* 1: 69-76.

Morrison, V. (1991) 'The impact of HIV upon injecting drug users: a longitudinal study', *AIDS Care* 3(2): 193-201.

Moss, A.R. and Bacchetti, P. (1989) 'Natural history of HIV infection', *AIDS* 3: 55-61.

Panos Institute (1990) *Triple Jeopardy: Women and AIDS*, London: Panos Publications.

Rhoads, J.L., Wright, C., Redfield, R.R. and Burke, D.S. (1987) 'Chronic vaginal candidiasis in women with human immunodeficiency virus infection', *Journal of the American Medical Association* 257: 3105-7.

Robertson, J.R., Bucknall, A.B.V., Welsby, P.D., Roberts, J.J.K., Inglis, J.M., Peutherer, J.F. and Brettle, R.P. (1986) 'Epidemic of AIDS-related virus (HTLV-III/LAV) infection among intravenous drug abusers', *British Medical Journal* 292: 527-9.

Robertson, J.R., Skidmore, C.A., Roberts, J.J.K. (1988) 'HIV infection in intravenous drug users: a follow-up study indicating change in risk-taking behaviour', *British Journal of Addiction* 83: 387-91.

Rothenberg, R., Woelfel, M., Stoneburner, R., Milberg, J., Parker, R. and Truman, B. (1987) 'Survival with the acquired immunodeficiency syndrome', *New England Journal of Medicine* 317: 1297-302.

Rutherford, G.W., Lifson, A.R., Hessol, N.A., Darrow, W.W., O'Malley, P.M., Buchbinder, S.P., Barnhart, J.L., Bodecker, T.W., Cannon, L., Doll, L.S., Holmberg, S.D., Harrison, J.S., Rogers, M.F., Werdegar, D. and Jaffe, H.W. (1990) 'Course of HIV-1 infection in a cohort of homosexual and bisexual men: an 11-year follow-up study', *British Medical Journal* 301: 1183-8.

Sato, P.A., Chin, J., Mann, J.M. (1989) 'Review of AIDS and HIV infection: global epidemiology and statistics', *AIDS* 3 (suppl. 1): 5301-7.

Willocks, L., Cowan, S.M., Brettle, R.P., MacCallum, L.R., McHardy, S. and Richardson, A. (1991) 'Natural history of early HIV infection in Scottish women'. Paper presented at VIIth International Conference on AIDS, Florence.

World Health Organisation (1990) 'AIDS and the status of women – challenges and perspectives for the 1990s', *WHO Features* No. 149, Geneva: World Health Organisation.

World Health Organisation (1991) Global Programme on AIDS.

2 Social issues
An overview

Joy Barlow

During the early years of the HIV/AIDS epidemic, all that was written and discussed about AIDS and its implications was drawn from the experiences of men who had sex with men. More recently, several books highlighting the issues for women have been published, (e.g. Richardson 1988, Rieder and Ruppelt 1989) and conferences around the topic of Women and AIDS have been organised. However, there has been very little analysis of the experience of women who are antibody positive or who have AIDS and there is still only a small voice heard from those women who are most profoundly affected by the virus.

As with so many other societal issues, we are in danger of extrapolating from the male situation to the female, and this is neither tenable nor indeed possible. Women's access to health care, the support systems available to them, their ability to make changes in their sex lives and their reactions to physical decline and disfigurement, are likely to be different from men's.

Social implications of HIV for women cannot be examined in isolation from the position of women in society. For so many women who are infected and affected, their position is characterised by financial and emotional dependence, which is reinforced by the legal system, the health care system and social services.

It is important to remember that in our society the adult who is powerless and dependent is regarded as having brought it upon her or himself. In the HIV/AIDS situation this is of crucial importance. It is therefore essential that those most closely involved are empowered to speak out and explain their own situations. Feelings of impotence and powerlessness must be dispelled by advocacy groups joining with and standing alongside HIV positive women, not speaking for them, but with them, so that their voices are heard more loudly.

When information about AIDS first became available, certain types of behaviour were identified as being risky, and the sexual partners of those indulging in that risky behaviour were seen to be at risk of infection with

HIV. Thus the female partners of injecting drug users and those of bisexual men were identified as were the female partners of those men infected because of contaminated blood products, e.g. men with haemophilia. A small number of women were infected by artificial insemination and some through blood transfusion. Women were also infected by their own injecting drug use.

Since it has been recognised that HIV is spreading within the general population, it has become inappropriate to focus only on partners of those involved in certain types of risk activity. It is behaviour that puts people at risk of HIV infection, and behaviour is the responsibility of everyone.

Apart from women who are infected themselves, HIV and AIDS affect women in many and varied ways. Women are affected as mothers, partners, siblings, carers and service providers to those with HIV infection and AIDS. At present the virus and its attendant problems may disproportionately affect those women least able to bear the burden. Women will often be the mainstay of families already disadvantaged by poverty and deprivation, families whose lives may be characterised by poor housing, poor educational opportunity, difficult family relationships and problems with chemical dependency.

Women living with HIV in the community will usually bear the responsibility for child care, housekeeping, health and social work department appointments, *and* their own illness, as well as the illness of partner, possibly children and other family members. Often their own needs are the least well met.

All infected women will suffer the discrimination, stigmatisation and marginalisation which the knowledge of HIV infection brings. There are also specific implications for women with regard to treatment options: few women, for example, get the opportunity to enter drug treatment programmes. Women (no less than men) have to deal with the reactions of employers, family and friends. Safer drug use and safer sex are difficult strategies to identify with and to adopt if self-esteem is very low. Women with HIV infection are also particularly affected by feelings of depression, anxiety, profound grief, the physical effects of the condition and the difficulties of finding support (Local Authority Officer Working Group 1989). In addition, if women are told that they cannot possibly have HIV infection, as this is an infection caused by homosexual promiscuity, then it is very difficult for them to identify their needs for services and support.

ISOLATION

People with HIV infection often become socially isolated due to the reactions of others which may be based upon misinformation and media hype. They also may not wish to mix socially because they feel too upset or embarrassed about their physical appearance. Women may be affected by this more than men. The social proscriptions and myths about women's appearance and physical condition cause many aspects of women's bodies, well or ill, to become sources of discomfort, pain or sorrow to them. We are either too fat or too thin!

It is of fundamental importance that women get useful information about their bodies. We need to challenge the attitudes that frequently lead women to be valued largely for their appearance and youth. Women living with HIV or AIDS are usually young but are growing old very quickly.

ANXIETY AND DEPRESSION

The anxiety and depression felt by many women living with HIV and AIDS can be severe and long-lasting and will have implications for the way they behave. They have a number of fears related to their illness including dying a slow, painful death isolated from the people they know and care about. Anxiety and depression are exacerbated by poor self-image, lack of fiscal resources and the lack of opportunities to make choices which disproportionately affect all women in society. Feelings of anxiety and rejection are also created by misinformed media presentations and television programmes.

Heightened anxiety may develop into a retreat into the defence mechanism of denial, into preoccupation with maintaining the health of others and into inertia. Women seeking assistance may find themselves uncertain as to how to proceed. They may be hindered by a lack of available information specific to their concerns and an absence of obvious sources of information.

PROFOUND GRIEF

Feelings of profound grief are experienced by everyone affected by HIV infection. This is brought about by a loss of health, body image, sexuality and reproductive potential. Most people with HIV infection are concerned about the question of procreation, an issue which often concerns those who face terminal illness. It is not unusual for a person infected by HIV or AIDS and his/her partner or spouse to have an overwhelming desire to leave behind some creation, and a child symbolises this need. A woman may regard becoming a mother as an important aspect of how she sees herself and her future, reinforced by societal influences; motherhood may enhance self-esteem or may be culturally expected.

OTHER FEELINGS

A host of other feelings are experienced by women. Mothers of infected children experience guilt and anguish about their other children, such as when they should be told, and what is their future. In the early days some women suffered abrupt and unsupported diagnoses, which continue to affect their lives. For many there is still the feeling of a lack of a natural community in which to find appropriate support. Society's assumptions about the role of women are instrumental in creating feelings of failure and impotence, yet society still places great responsibility on the position of women. The assumption that women have responsibility for the control of sex and contraception lays an added burden on women who are known to be sero-positive or believe themselves to be at risk.

WOMEN WITH HIV INFECTION

Whilst all members of society must recognise their responsibility with regard to HIV and AIDS, there are still some women who are more likely to be infected.

The first of these are women who have been, or continue to be, injecting drug users. These women may be hard to reach in order to deliver the best form of care and their inaccessibility is understandable since society's perception of these women is that they have rejected their female role. Society continues to be profoundly shocked by women who are seen to have consciously stepped outside accepted boundaries. Drug injecting women have gone against society's perceived role of women as servicers and nurturers. They often find themselves stigmatised and isolated, with few supportive networks and a lack of family support. Their low self-esteem and self-perception cause them to shy away from asking for help, even if help is available. They withdraw from society and do not present to services out of fear of further condemnation. Most drug users, male or female, have difficulties relating to what they see as authority, and their experience of medical and social services may be negative.

Safer sex strategies rely to a great extent upon the individual having some awareness and concern about themselves as sexual beings. Many female drug injectors have suffered sexual abuse, and therefore their image of themselves as sexual is almost non-existent. Both sex and needle risks may come from a drug-injecting partner who may be recalcitrant in acknowledging his own risk and in taking responsibility. Women who inject have few resources except those individuals who work or live alongside them; yet these women may be responsible for children, for keeping a home together and for all the responsibilities carried by any woman in society.

Women who become infected by men who have sex with men will also experience feelings of loss of self-esteem, guilt and fear. They have the two-fold consideration of disclosure of information about the lover's sex life as well as their own. The guilt and inadequacy felt by many women who discover their sexual partner's sexual preference can be very damaging. The effect of an undisclosed sexual relationship may devastate any relationship, but to learn that the relationship has been with another man may be more difficult to accept.

The partners of haemophiliac men infected with HIV are faced with yet another set of health problems, as well as those presented by haemophilia, and there is also the risk that they might become infected themselves. Mothers of haemophiliac boys may feel guilty because, not only are they responsible genetically for their son's condition, but they may also have been the person who injected the contaminated blood product. There is also the constant fear that, although the risk of contaminated blood products is now very small, a mother may still put her son at risk. Yet he needs this blood product in order to stay alive. A national campaign which focuses on sexual behaviour may ring very hollow to mothers of haemophiliac boys.

Women affected by haemophilia in their family may feel stigmatised, isolated and discriminated against because of society's reaction to HIV (Markova and Forbes 1984; Markova and Wilkie 1987).

Haemophiliac men and their partners are now very reluctant to admit that they suffer from haemophilia because of its associations with AIDS. The men have repeatedly emphasised that public attitudes and prejudice with respect to their haemophilia are often more unbearable than the disease itself.

WOMEN FROM ETHNIC MINORITIES

Many women from minority backgrounds will be affected by religious and social proscriptions, due to certain fundamentalist traditions within their own cultures or tribal customs. Women from sub-Saharan Africa tend to present very late for help at services in London because of such constraints (Positively Women, personal communication 1991). Some women may find it difficult to get appropriate information because of their lack of knowledge of English, and the unavailability of services in their own language. Some may have had to rely on their partners' knowledge of English.

The National Health Service and Social Services in general still discriminate against women from ethnic backgrounds. For these women HIV/AIDS is just another inequality. Women from ethnic backgrounds recognise that society often believes that their culture is their problem. It is because they are Black, for example, that they have problems, not that society's attitude towards them may be problematic. They are also deeply affected by myths about the origin of AIDS. The idea that AIDS originated in Africa has brought further discrimination to Black and other ethnic groups. In 1991, the National Blood Transfusion Service was still asking whether an individual had had sex with someone from Africa. A similar question relating to a person from the USA was not asked.

With regard to HIV and AIDS prevention material, it is not good enough to have simple translations from the English language. All resources should include images which are multiculturally acceptable. It is not always recognised that some languages do not have corresponding words for English ones, and even some concepts are difficult to translate. There has been justified criticism from some Black and Asian HIV/AIDS workers about the stereotypical nature of leaflets and posters targeted at ethnic minority women.

LESBIAN WOMEN

Since the beginning of the epidemic, lesbians have been affected as workers in the caring professions, they have been affected by AIDS through the related deaths of gay men they know and they have been affected by the strengthening of anti-gay feeling.

Until recently, it was erroneously believed that lesbian women were not affected sexually by HIV and AIDS and safer sex practices and HIV risks are not something that most lesbians in Britain have thought about. First, it was believed that they would not get AIDS, and second, lesbians, like most women, do not find it easy to talk about sex. Lesbian women may find this even more difficult than heterosexual women as they are not used to having to think about protection against infection or prevention of pregnancy. Although the risk of HIV infection from sex between women is very small it is important for lesbians to look at what they do, how they do it and with whom they do it, just like everyone else – 'Low risk isn't no risk' (London Lesbian and Gay Switchboard 1990).

Some lesbians inject drugs and share equipment. Some lesbians may have sex with men for a living or other reasons. Some have or want to have children. Those who choose donor insemination face potential risks. If women make private arrangements for this, and they may have to do so, it is important that they have information about the need for HIV testing of donors. If lesbian women choose to become pregnant by heterosexual sex, then the same precautions apply.

There have been two published cases of women becoming infected with HIV through sex with women (Chu *et al.* 1990). In both cases, the sexual activities involved included the exchange of blood. HIV infection among lesbian women is not recorded separately in published statistics and lesbian women may be reluctant to acknowledge their sexual orientation to their doctor. The number of women infected by sex with women may therefore be underestimated.

Just like everyone else, lesbian women need to take care of themselves. However, they may find it difficult to access services and if they become ill they may experience special problems, given that the health care system is designed for and administered by a predominantly heterosexual population. There may be a lack of recognition of their relationships, and this may lead to isolation and depression (Lisa Power, personal communication 1991).

TEENAGE GIRLS

Perhaps one of the most difficult groups for whom to make HIV/AIDS prevention relevant are those teenage girls who are becoming sexually active in the age of AIDS.

On the one hand teenagers of both sexes are subject to the 'hard sell' of advertising which seduces and cajoles the recipient into the belief that sex sells and buys everything. From the comparatively innocuous adverts for denim jeans to the tabloid press Page Three girls, sex is everywhere. On the other hand, there is an enormous amount of talk and discussion with regard to HIV/AIDS prevention, some of which may give the impression that sex is now an activity which kills. Sexually active teenage girls must be very confused.

The same arguments about teenage girls and HIV/AIDS prevention can be applied to safer sex practices which may reduce the risk of pregnancy. Emotions are highly charged, and behaviour hinges on wanting to have sex, being ready to have sex, and being able to practice safer sex and/or contraception at the same time.

Britain has not wholeheartedly recognised the educational needs of young people in this area. Taboos and prejudices still abound (Bury 1991). Yet in Sweden, for example, schoolgirls who are in their early teens are taught to place a condom over a model of an erect penis.

For the child educated in the 1980s and 1990s, AIDS is as much a part of social reality as Chernobyl, drug addiction and Eastenders. Education for prevention must recognise HIV and AIDS as a social reality.

WOMEN AS CARERS

Caring is an activity which is seen as natural for women. Traditionally women have been seen as care givers, because of their 'inherent capacity to nurture others' (Nash 1990). Consequently, women are expected to care yet may be ill-resourced and unsupported themselves. 'Invisible' caring by women is already a feature of life in those communities profoundly affected by HIV (Ramsay and Wilson 1990).

'Community care', as defined in the provision of the National Health Service and Community Care Act (1990), includes the promotion of domiciliary and day services to encourage people to live in their own homes while giving high priority to supporting carers. In Chapter 3 of the White Paper 'Caring for People', which provided the background to the Act, the important role of the informal carer was highlighted (Department of Health and Social Security 1989). Thus, in the age of 'Community Care', family caring such as that described above will be the expected mode of delivery of a great deal of care. The burden laid upon some families will be immense, and will only be sustained by sensitively delivered resources from statutory authorities.

In their experience of care, women may feel pain and anger after finding out about the sexual orientation or lifestyle of their partner or child. Mothers may feel unvoiced pain when they become the sounding board for their child's anger and frustration. Care also involves feelings such as the uncertainty of life expectancy, isolation, lack of support and fear of infectivity. Care is also about work. Women are seen as being able to cope; they are rarely asked what help and support they need to enable them to do the job of caring. A woman may be pressurised into giving up paid work in order to care for someone with HIV infection.

Caring for children will be very distressing. For an HIV positive mother, there is concern not only about her own health and possible impending death, but also about the health of her child and its life expectancy, as well as the future of sibling brothers and sisters.

It is with respect to the care of children, and the future of families, that the two concepts of empowerment and protection have to be faced. Whilst enabling a woman to care for her children until she can no longer do so, it must be recognised that society will expect the protection of children to be paramount. The constant tension between the two concepts will be held by all the caring professions, and they will need support in order to carry that tension.

In spite of the many difficulties for women that have been described, there have been some very positive responses. Women whose psychological identities are forged out of concern for their own survival, need not give up their capacity for warmth, emotionality and nurturing. Women need not stop being tender, compassionate or concerned with the feelings of others; they can start being tender and compassionate with themselves as well. Recently the increased activity of groups recognising the special needs of women, such as Positively Women and the Scottish Women and HIV/AIDS Network, has given hope for the future. These organisations recognise that women's interests may have been ignored, misunderstood and neglected, and that these attitudes should be challenged.

The sentiments expressed in this quotation from a French social scientist should motivate us all:

> To those women who say we cannot resist, who say it is too much to ask that we resist, I would say that women have always resisted. As part of their daily efforts to attain self-esteem and survival, women have always fought back.
>
> (Anyon 1984:85)

REFERENCES

Anyon, J. (1984) 'Interactions of gender and class: accommodation and resistance by working-class and affluent females to contradictory sex role ideology', *Journal of Education* 166: 79-85.

Bury, J.K. (1991) 'Teenage sexual behaviour and the impact of AIDS', *Health Education Journal* 50: 43-9.

Chu, S.Y., Buchler, J.W., Fleming, P.L. and Berkelman, R.L. (1990) 'Epidemiology of reported cases of AIDS in lesbians, United States 1980-89', *American Journal of Public Health* 80: 1380-1.

Department of Health and Social Security (1989) *Caring for People: Community Care in the Next Decade and Beyond*, London: HMSO.

Local Authority Officer Working Group (1989) *Women, Children and HIV*, Association of Metropolitan Authorities.

London Lesbian and Gay Switchboard (1990) *Lesbians, HIV and Safer Sex – Low Risk isn't No Risk*, London: Lesbian and Gay Switchboard Ltd.

Markova, I. and Forbes, C.D. (1984) 'Coping with haemophilia', *International Review of Applied Psychology* 33: 457-77.

Markova, I. and Wilkie, P. (1987) 'Representations, concepts and social change: the phenomenon of AIDS', *Journal for the Theory of Social Behaviour* 17: 4.

Nash, P. (1990) 'Caring for people with HIV/AIDS: a professional perspective', in *Women Talking About AIDS*, London: AVERT.

Ramsay, J. and Wilson, J. (1990) 'Invisible caring in Edinburgh', in S. Henderson (ed.) *Women, HIV and Drugs*, London: I. S. D. D.

Richardson, D. (1988) *Women and the AIDS Crisis*, London: Pandora.

Rieder, I. and Ruppelt, P. (eds) (1989) *Matters of Life and Death: Women Speak About AIDS*, London: Virago.

3   Reflections on women and HIV/AIDS in New York City and the United States

Edith Springer

FRAMING THE PROBLEM

AIDS cases in women represent about 10 per cent of the total AIDS cases in the United States (see Table 3.1). In New York City women represent about 15 per cent of the total cases (see Table 3.2). Since there are fewer infected women than men there is less information available about how HIV affects women. Research studies generally exclude women and drug users by design so that little data is available for those treating HIV-infected women's medical problems. On a psychosocial level, women are more isolated and have fewer supports and services available to them which are tailored to their needs; they have to integrate themselves into services created for men.

The racial/ethnic imbalance in the statistics is startling. Minorities, predominantly Black and Hispanic women, are over-represented while White women are under-represented. Minority women are the poorest women in the United States and they are shouldering a greater burden with HIV/AIDS. In a racist country, such as the United States, minority groups suffer from all kinds of discrimination and deprivation, particularly economic, vocational and educational deprivation, which puts them at an extreme disadvantage in society. Medical care for the poor is hard to access and is often of questionable quality. Many are now homeless, a status from which it is almost impossible to recover, particularly in New York City where housing for the poor is unavailable. Minorities are shouldering the major bulk of the paediatric AIDS cases. In New York State 54 per cent of paediatric cases are Black, 35 per cent are Hispanic, while only 11 per cent are White. In the US 56 per cent of paediatric cases are Black, 26 per cent are Hispanic, while 21 per cent are White. In some neighbourhoods, such as Harlem, one senses an entire age group is missing – men and women aged 20–40 years – a group which has already died.

The age groups of women affected by HIV (Table 3.1) illustrate that the largest group of women are in the 25–44 age group, the childbearing years,

Table 3.1 Targeted surveillance information, USA

Adult AIDS cases to June 1991 (CDC)	179,694	
Paediatric AIDS cases	3,140	
Total	182,834	
Adult women		
Total cases	18,201	(10%)
By risk factor		
IVDU	9,623	(51%)
Haemophilia/coag.	38	(0%)
Heterosexual cont.	6,035	(33%)
Sex with IVDU	3,763	
Sex with bisexual male	567	
Sex with person with haem.	86	
Born in pattern II country*	623	
Sex with person born in pattern II country*	66	
Sex with transfusion recipient	134	
Sex with HIV+, unspecified	797	
Receipt of blood transfusion tissue	1,554	(9%)
Undetermined/Other	1,311	(7%)
By age at diagnosis		
Under 5	1,236	(6%)
5–12	215	(1%)
13–19	183	(1%)
20–24	1,213	(6%)
25–29	3,583	(18%)
30–34	4,824	(25%)
35–39	3,694	(19%)
40–44	1,877	(10%)
45–49	906	(5%)
50–54	572	(3%)
55–59	413	(2%)
60–64	325	(2%)
65 and older	611	(3%)
By ethnicity		
White	4,764	
Black	9,496	
Hispanic	3,766	
Asian/Pacific Is.	93	
American Indian/Alaskan	34	

*Pattern II country: countries where extensive spread of HIV infection probably began in the mid- to late 1970s and is found predominantly in sexually active heterosexuals, e.g. sub-Saharan Africa and some parts of the Caribbean.
Source: US Department of Health and Human Services, 1991

with the result that the rate of paediatric cases from perinatal transmission is high. There are 3,140 paediatric cases in the US as of June 1991. Of these cases, 83 per cent resulted from perinatal transmission.

New York State paediatric cases (under age 13) indicate that in 58 per

Table 3.2 Targeted surveillance information, New York City

Total cases to June 1991	31,541	
Total female cases	4,828	(15%)
Female cases by risk factor		
IVDU	2,952	(61%)
Haemophiliac	2	(0%)
Heterosexual contact	1,228	(25%)
Foreign born	148	(3%)
Transfusion	77	(2%)
Undetermined	421	(9%)
Paediatric (under 13)	411	(8%)
Female cases by race/ethnicity		
White	667	
Black	2,510	
Hispanic	1,609	
Other/missing	25	

Source: New York State Department of Health, 1991

cent of the cases the mother was an injecting drug user and in another 19 per cent of the cases the mother had had sex with an injecting drug user. There are a total of 733 paediatric cases in New York State, 648 of whom are in New York City.

Injecting drug use is still the most frequent cause of infection, with 51 per cent of the US AIDS cases and 57 per cent of the New York City cases resulting from equipment sharing. The US and NYC have chosen to withhold the key interventions which would have helped to stop such transmission, i.e. syringe distribution/exchange, drug treatment on demand, massive outreach programs. Women are still out there sharing equipment and getting infected.

WHO ARE THE WOMEN WITH HIV/AIDS IN NEW YORK CITY?

While HIV/AIDS has befallen women from all races, classes and walks of life, the bulk of the women being infected are poor minority women. The link is injecting drug use and the sharing of injection equipment due to the unavailability of sterile equipment. In eleven states in the US including New York, New Jersey and Connecticut, it is illegal to possess a hypodermic syringe without a prescription from a physician. These states have 84 per cent of the injecting drug-related AIDS cases in the nation. While the majority of cases in women result directly from the women's injecting drug use, the second largest group becoming infected are the sex partners of injecting drug users. Injecting drug use is the link between women and HIV and perinatal transmission.

In many urban areas in the United States, and particularly in parts of New York City, crack cocaine (cocaine hydrochloride, which is free-based and sold in rock form which can be smoked in a pipe) has overtaken heroin as the drug of choice. It is seen in West and Central Harlem, the Lower East Side of Manhattan, the South Bronx, parts of Brooklyn and Queens. Many former injecting drug users are now smoking crack. Some are still injecting heroin as well, particularly to help with the rebound from crack which is very brutal and often involves suicidal depression. Many of the minority women in these neighbourhoods have adopted crack as their first drug of use while many others have switched from heroin. Some switched from heroin thinking smoking crack would reduce their risk of HIV infection, since HIV is not transmitted through pipe stems. However, crack houses, or places for buying and using crack and for buying and selling sex, sprang up and crack users, often very young pre-teenagers, began selling sex for bowls of crack. The cheapest dose of crack in New York costs $3 and the cheapest sex act costs the same in a crack house. This crack epidemic has caused an epidemic in sexually transmitted diseases, with syphilis up 600 per cent and gonorrhoea up 400 per cent in New York City (New York City Department of Health 1990). Sexually transmitted diseases which involve genital lesions have been found to increase the risk of HIV transmission (e.g. Plummer *et al.* 1988). Needless to say, the sex that goes on in crack houses is not safe sex but unprotected sex. The New York City Department of Health expects the next wave of AIDS cases to be in adolescents who use crack and sell sex.

There are very few treatment slots for those with crack problems – the largest treatment capacity in New York offers methadone maintenance which is not appropriate for crack users. The therapeutic communities have only a few thousand slots in the entire state of New York and these are for all types of drug users. We don't know how to treat crack problems and traditional treatment programmes appear to be averse to experimenting with alternative modes of treatment, such as acupuncture and other holistic remedies which show promise. The drug treatment system has about 50,000 slots throughout the state. There are an estimated 260,000 needle users and about 300,000–500,000 crack users competing for those 50,000 treatment slots. Treatment tends to be judgemental, sadistic, designed for men and oblivious to the special needs of women. Success rates in treatment are generally below 10 per cent. Treatment, much touted as the answer to the drug-related AIDS problem, is no answer to anything at all, not even drug problems.

THE UNITED STATES' 'WAR ON DRUGS'

Nothing has hindered the work of AIDS prevention with drug users more than the ill-conceived, moralistic 'War on Drugs'. Far from being a public health response to a public health issue, the War on Drugs has caused the most harmful drugs, such as crack, to be readily available, of high quality and cheap, but the least harmful drugs, such as marijuana and pure heroin, to be expensive and hard to get. Drugs and drug users are now universally accepted evils and the government has set the tone for more discrimination and sadistic treatment of drug users. Most drug users end up in the correctional system. It has been estimated that 70 per cent of people in jails and prisons in the US are there for drug-related crimes. The cost of incarcerating so many people is astounding, particularly when drug treatment is far cheaper. In New York City, for example, it costs $25,000 to keep a person in jail for a year; it costs only $15,000 to keep that same person in a residential therapeutic community where they receive treatment and education in addition to room and board.

The War on Drugs has caused drug users more fear, more arrests, more incarcerations, more disruption of families, more economic ruin and home-lessness, more stigma and more hiding underground. This is devastating to a population which needs contact with helping services yet runs from them for fear of maltreatment. The War on Drugs is also incredibly expensive and has taken funds away from AIDS and other important issues. All the money is going to interdiction even though history shows us that prohibition doesn't work. It seems as though America needed a new enemy after detente and our new friendship with the Soviets, and we picked drugs and drug users as the enemy.

Because of the War on Drugs mentality, interventions which have been proven to work against HIV, such as syringe exchanges, maintenance of long-term drug users on their drugs of choice, and improvement and expan-sion of drug treatment services, have been ignored. Many people believe that the US government is thrilled to see its gay and drug using minority popula-tions being wiped out. The minority community refers to it as genocide. Harm reduction models, so successful in England, Scotland and other countries, are despised by the powers in charge. The former New York City Commissioner of Health, Woodrow Myers, a middle-class black man, closed New York's needle exchange pilot experiment after ten months, saying that drug users must face the consequences of their behaviour. He said this even though poor black people are getting wiped out by HIV.

AIDS IN WOMEN: LACK OF RECOGNITION AND SHORTER SURVIVAL

From the beginning of the epidemic, the epidemiological definition of AIDS created by the Centers for Disease Control (CDC) has excluded many severely immunocompromised HIV positive women from receiving an AIDS diagnosis and thus being counted in the statistics. Although the definition of AIDS has been broadened over time, it still does not reflect the clinical manifestations observed in women. Outside of New York City, where doctors may be less aware that AIDS can affect women, many conditions such as *Pneumocystis carinii* pneumonia, a marker of AIDS in men, may go overlooked in women. Deaths from respiratory infections have dramatically risen in young women in New York City during the 1980s. Many of these women received inappropriate treatment because the physicians did not look for HIV (New York State Department of Health AIDS Institute 1990).

However, since the definition of AIDS by the Centers for Disease Control has only focused on men, women with, for example, pelvic inflammatory disease who are HIV infected, are denied an AIDS diagnosis, leaving them unable to apply for benefits they need and deserve, but cannot obtain without an AIDS diagnosis. Eleven years into the epidemic in the US and the CDC is now telling us they will revise this definition 'in a couple of months'.

Since the start of the epidemic, women have lived the shortest time from AIDS diagnosis to death (see Chapter 1). Minority women have the shortest time of all.

Poor minority women are unlikely to be receiving ongoing preventive medical care and they are also unlikely to go to see a doctor when they are sick. Often they do not enter the health care system until they are even further along in their disease when treatments are even less effective.

ABANDONMENT, ISOLATION AND SUPPORT

Women often stick by their men through HIV infection, illness and death. Men often abandon their women when they become HIV infected or ill. Women may be left ill with children to care for, some of whom are also ill. Many extended family systems are taking care of entire families with AIDS and many elderly grandmothers and aunts are caring for family members. We often forget about all the women affected by AIDS who may not be infected with HIV.

Until recently there were almost no support groups for women with HIV in New York City. Now there are several, although nowhere near a sufficient number for the women who need them. Women who are ill or burdened with children and without another caretaker, cannot travel great distances to attend these groups.

Many of the AIDS organisations and services are frequented almost exclusively by men, many of them gay men, and women often feel uncomfortable in those settings. Often racial/ethnic and class differences keep poor minority women from participating in available services. They feel uncomfortable that they have no money, their clothes are shabby, and they have nothing in common with the other participants. Women with HIV/AIDS are therefore far more isolated than men and have fewer services available to them.

PROSTITUTION, DRUGS AND HIV

Prostitutes have been badly maligned in this epidemic. All prostitutes are branded as 'vectors of transmission' who are giving AIDS to their 'johns'. Nothing could be further from the truth (see e.g., Plant 1990). The majority of prostitutes, that is, those who are not drug users, have the same infection rates as the general population of women. It is needle-using women who sell sex who have high seroprevalence rates. Most of these women began selling sex to finance their drug habits; a guaranteed income or vocational training or a medical supply of drugs would eliminate their need to sell sex.

Drug-using women (regardless of their drug of choice) who sell sex often lead 'double lives', hiding both their drug use and their prostitution from their families. This further impedes HIV risk-reduction activities and seeking help.

Drug-using women are seen as evil vectors of transmission who give HIV to their babies. They are seen as evil people who addict their babies to drugs before they are born. In the US women are only valued as baby factories; the woman herself is not considered important. Thus, in Florida, women who deliver babies with drugs in their urine are arrested and their children are taken from them. In New York City, hearings are held at birth to determine if the child should be taken into care. Women are not valued as human beings and citizens, only as receptacles for semen and manufacturers of babies, who are often referred to as the 'innocent victims of AIDS'. Are the mothers not innocent victims?

PHYSICAL AND SEXUAL ABUSE IN WOMEN AS A BARRIER TO PREVENTION

Among drug-using women the rates of sexual abuse (as children and as adults) and physical abuse, including spouse abuse, are extremely high (see e.g., Worth 1990). Women often have little power in their sexual relationships. Bargaining for risk-reduction practices such as condom use can lead to a beating and still no possibility of preventing HIV infection. In one drug treatment programme over 70 per cent of the women indicated past histories of sexual and physical abuse (Daytop Village Therapeutic Community, personal communication 1986). Many minority women who wish to use condoms are unable to do so because their male partners control when and how they have sex, and birth control is avoided by macho males who want to prove their virility by making children.

There is no sexual barrier that women can use without men's co-operation. This leaves a woman with no other technology or device or method to protect herself beyond saying 'no', which in some cases can lead to assault by her man.

PERCEPTION OF GENOCIDE IN MINORITY COMMUNITIES

While the White professionals' response to HIV perinatal transmission is to advise minority women to 'postpone pregnancy' and abort if they are HIV positive, the minority community perceives that genocide is being perpetrated on it. Their response to this is to make more babies to try to keep their race from dying out.

The chances of an infected mother passing the virus on to her child is believed to be much lower than originally thought (see Chapter 4). The rates are now thought to be about 30 per cent in New York. To a minority family which is already in a group with high infant mortality and morbidity rates, these do not seem like bad odds. The problem is that one has to wait 15–18 months before the child can be tested to get a true picture of its HIV status (see Chapter 4). Many ignorant physicians in the US test the babies right away and tell the mother that the baby is infected.

When professionals say 'abort' and 'don't get pregnant' and clients respond by trying to get pregnant and not aborting, friction develops between the helpers and the clients. Professionals must learn to keep their own values and judgements to themselves and support clients by helping them accomplish their own goals, not those of the worker.

WOMEN'S CONNECTION TO CHILDREN: A DISADVANTAGE

Service providers neglect to take account of the fact that many of our minority women are the sole providers and caretakers for their children. The welfare system in New York is set up to link children and mothers and exclude fathers. A woman may receive public assistance just by virtue of being a mother of minor children whereas men have to have a disability to receive assistance. Often the mother must eject the man or he 'floats' around, staying out of the way so that she may receive benefits. Yet service providers do not provide child care so that women may avail themselves of services. Most residential drug treatment programmes discriminate against women with children by forcing women to give up their children in order to enter treatment. In the entire state of New York there are only about twenty-five spaces for women in drug treatment with their children. Many women who give up their children 'temporarily' to family members find that these relatives have gone to court and legally taken the children away while the mother was trying to rehabilitate herself in drug treatment.

Women are usually poorer than their male counterparts because they support the children while the men often take no economic responsibility for them. Women are also prevented from entering vocational programmes because there is no child care available: a vicious cycle.

SURVIVAL NEEDS OF UNDERCLASS WOMEN ARE NOT MET BY SOCIETY

Many of the women most vulnerable to HIV and those with HIV and AIDS are underclass women. They are dirt poor, often minority group members, who may or may not speak or be literate in English. The majority do not have housing of their own, if they have a shelter to live in at all. Their daily quest is for their survival needs and those of their children. Where to sleep tonight, what to eat, where to get money for drugs or food, where to find warm clothing for herself and her children, how to avoid the violence all around her – these are the survival needs they face every day. Trying to get them to focus on health promotion and AIDS prevention is a difficult task. It is a great fear of theirs, yet they feel helpless to do anything about it. In order to do real AIDS prevention work, we have to first meet these women's survival needs.

REFERENCES

New York City Department of Health (1990) personal communication.

New York State Department of Health (1991) *AIDS Surveillance Monthly Update for Cases Reported through June 1991*, Bureau of Communicable Disease Control.

New York State Department of Health AIDS Institute (1990) 'Women and the impact of the HIV/AIDS epidemic', *Focus on AIDS in New York State* 2(2): 1-2.

Plant, M. (ed.) (1990) *AIDS, Drugs and Prostitution*, London: Routledge.

Plummer, F., Cameron, W., Simonsen, N., Bosire, M., Maitha, G., Kreiss, J., Waiyaki, P., Ronald, A., Ndinya-Achola, J. and Ngugi, F. (1988) 'Co-factors in male-female transmission of HIV'. Paper presented at IVth International Conference on AIDS, Stockholm.

US Department of Health and Human Services (1991) *US AIDS Cases Reported through June 1991*, Atlanta, Georgia: Centers for Disease Control.

Worth, D. (1990) 'Sexual and physical abuse in childhood: a barrier to risk reduction in intravenous drug using women'. Paper presented at VIth International Conference on AIDS, San Francisco.

Part II

Contraception and pregnancy

4 Pregnancy, heterosexual transmission and contraception

Judy Bury

By the end of 1991, 1,952 women in the UK had been found to have antibodies to the human immunodeficiency virus. These are women who have come forward for HIV testing and there is general agreement (e.g. Peckham and Newell 1990) that they represent only a small proportion of the total number of women in the UK infected with HIV. More than 90 per cent of women who are known to be HIV positive are of child-bearing age (see Table 4.1) and many have not yet started or completed their families.

Anonymous antenatal screening tests carried out in 1991 found that only 1 in 16,000 pregnant women in the UK was infected with HIV but in some areas of London as many as 1 pregnant woman in 220 was infected (Medical Research Council 1991). In the same year it was found that the prevalence of HIV infection in women who had just given birth in Edinburgh was 2.5 per 1,000, in Dundee 1.4 per 1,000 and in Aberdeen 0.7 per 1,000 (Tappin *et al.* 1991). A similar study carried out in London provides evidence of a rising HIV prevalence among childbearing women; the prevalence of HIV infection in recently delivered mothers in inner London had risen from

Table 4.1 Age distribution of HIV-antibody positive women at time of test: UK up to 31.12.90

Age group	No. of women with HIV infection*
0–14	88 (6%)
15–24	584 (38%)
25–34	674 (44%)
35–44	133 (9%)
45–54	26 (2%)
55 or over	22 (1%)
Total	1,527

* Table excludes 102 women where age was not stated.
Source: Adapted from *Communicable Disease Report* (1991) 1(10): 46

1 in 2,000 in 1988–9 to 1 in 500 in the first three months of 1991 (Ades *et al.* 1991).

The issue of HIV infection and childbearing has been surrounded by confusion and misinformation with the result that it has sometimes been difficult for women with HIV infection, and other women at risk of infection, to obtain accurate information and advice about pregnancy, about the risks of heterosexual transmission and about the suitability of different methods of contraception for them.

PREGNANCY

In discussing the risks of pregnancy for women with HIV infection there are four main issues to consider: the effect of pregnancy on the progression of HIV disease; the effect of HIV infection on the outcome of pregnancy; the risk of materno-fetal transmission of HIV infection; and the risk of transmitting HIV through breast feeding. Much of the confusion about pregnancy and HIV infection has been caused by the results of early studies and this will be discussed. The implications of the risks of pregnancy for counselling women with HIV infection will also be considered.

Early studies

During the early 1980s, studies from the United States suggested that pregnancy was dangerous for women with HIV infection as it appeared to increase the risk of progression to AIDS. These studies (e.g. Scott 1984) were carried out before testing for HIV antibodies was available. Their starting point therefore, was not women with HIV infection but babies who developed AIDS, whose mothers were then followed up. It seemed that pregnancy itself acted as a co-factor for the development of AIDS in an infected woman and, at that stage, this was thought to be due to the known immunosuppressant effect of pregnancy.

Testing for HIV antibodies became available in 1985 and since then it has been possible to follow HIV positive women through their pregnancies to see what effect the pregnancy has on the progress of the mother's HIV disease and also what effect HIV infection has on the outcome of pregnancy.

Pregnancy and the progression of HIV disease

An Edinburgh study carried out in 1987 followed 28 HIV positive asymptomatic women through their pregnancies and found that the pregnancy had no deleterious effect on their health or on their immune system (MacCallum 1988). Since then other studies have confirmed these findings (see Schoenbaum *et al.* 1988) and the current view is that pregnancy does not affect the progression of HIV disease in women who are still asymptomatic and whose immune system is still intact.

However, once HIV disease has progressed to the stage where the woman's immune system has been compromised, pregnancy may cause more rapid progression of the disease. It is not yet clear whether terminating the pregnancy would protect the woman from this danger (Minkoff 1987).

Although most recent studies have been reassuring about the risks of pregnancy, Minkoff (1987) has pointed out that pregnancy may mask the early symptoms of HIV disease such as tiredness and breathlessness and that, if a woman develops AIDS during pregnancy, treatment may be more difficult as some of the useful drugs might harm the fetus.

HIV infection and the outcome of pregnancy

Studies in Edinburgh and New York in 1987 found that women with HIV infection who were still well fared no worse during their pregnancies than women in similar circumstances (that is, drug users or partners of drug users) who were not HIV infected (Johnstone *et al.* 1988, Selwyn *et al.* 1989). Although *all* these women experienced many complications of pregnancy, the authors concluded that HIV infection does not increase the risk of having a miscarriage, a stillbirth, a premature baby or a baby of low birthweight.

The Edinburgh authors emphasise that it is not yet known if symptomatic HIV infection is more likely to affect the outcome of pregnancy (Johnstone *et al.* 1988). For example, a study in Zaire found that infants born to HIV infected women, many of whom were at an advanced stage in the disease, were more likely to be premature and of low birthweight and to have a higher neonatal mortality rate than infants of seronegative mothers (Ryder *et al.* 1989).

Materno-fetal transmission of HIV infection

The possibility that HIV infection might pass from a mother to her baby during pregnancy was recognised at an early stage in the epidemic, even before the causative infective agent had been identified (e.g. Scott *et al.* 1984). The virus can cross the placenta as early as 20 weeks of pregnancy and the factors that determine whether or not this occurs are still uncertain. A recent study has suggested that transmission of HIV may also occur close to or at the time of delivery (Ehrnst *et al.* 1991). Although vaginal delivery may increase the risk of transmission (Chiodo *et al.* 1986) Caesarian section does not appear to protect the fetus from infection (e.g. Lifson and Rogers 1986).

The studies during the early 1980s already referred to (p. 44) suggested a rate of transmission of about 50 per cent but as we have seen these studies were hampered by the absence of tests for HIV antibodies, so that only symptomatic mothers and children could be identified. However, now that women with HIV infection can be identified, all their babies can be studied.

At present it is not possible to test reliably for the virus itself, so diagnosis of HIV infection depends on the presence of HIV antibodies. This makes the diagnosis of HIV infection in newborn babies difficult as all babies born to HIV positive mothers will have maternal HIV antibodies at birth. These maternal antibodies clear by 18 months so that if a baby is not infected, it will be HIV negative by 18 months. If the baby is infected, it will make its own antibodies to HIV, thus remaining HIV positive beyond 18 months. It is therefore not possible to know whether or not a baby is infected until it is 18 months of age. Other tests that may allow earlier diagnosis are being evaluated but are not yet available (Peckham and Newell 1990).

In a recent study of 600 babies born to HIV-infected mothers in ten European Centres, only 13 per cent had persistent HIV antibody after 18 months, suggesting a transmission rate of approximately 1 in 8, much lower than previously thought (European Collaborative Study 1991).

One important factor that seems to affect the risk of materno-fetal transmission is the health of the mother during pregnancy. In one study, infants born to mothers who had symptoms of HIV infection during pregnancy were nine times more likely to develop AIDS or AIDS-related complex than infants of mothers who were clinically well during pregnancy (Mok *et al.* 1987). The early studies which showed high rates of transmission of infection to the baby included many women who already had symptoms of HIV infection. In the recent European study which showed a low transmission rate, only 5 per cent of the mothers were symptomatic during pregnancy or by three months after birth (European Collaborative Study 1991).

It has been suggested that there may also be a greater risk of transmission at the time a woman becomes HIV antibody positive (seroconversion) – a time when there are a large number of viruses (HIV) in the bloodstream. Although this is still uncertain, this possibility has implications for those advising women without HIV infection but who have an HIV positive partner and who risk becoming infected at the time of conception or during pregnancy.

Reinterpretation of early studies

It is now easier to understand why early studies of mothers of babies who developed AIDS gave such misleading results. As we have seen, mothers who transmit HIV infection to their babies are more likely to be at an advanced stage of their disease and are therefore more likely to develop AIDS during or soon after the pregnancy. By studying only these women, it was inevitable that pregnancy would seem to be causing progression of the woman's HIV disease and that the risk of the baby being infected would be misleadingly high.

Although these studies have now been superseded, their impact remains. There continue to be reports of women being advised not to become pregnant or to have their pregnancy terminated because of the risk to their health. Women are also given misleading information about the possibility that their baby will be infected.

Counselling HIV positive women about pregnancy

It is now possible for a woman to be given more individual advice about the risk of pregnancy for her and her baby. If a woman has symptoms of HIV infection or has AIDS there is a substantial risk that the baby will be infected and that pregnancy will cause a more rapid progression of her illness. If she is asymptomatic, immunological and virological blood tests might give some clues about disease progression and the likelihood of imminent clinical deterioration (Anonymous 1988). If there is no evidence of severe damage to the immune system and clinical deterioration does not seem imminent, and if she is keen to have a baby, even knowing that the baby might be infected, it is probably better for her to have a baby sooner rather than later, as her health is less likely to be affected, the baby is less likely to be infected, and she is likely to have more years to spend with the baby before becoming ill herself.

In reality, an HIV-infected woman's decision about the future of her pregnancy will be determined by many factors other than the risk to her health and the health of her baby. She may wish to have a baby as it may be the only creative thing she has ever done. Knowledge of her HIV status and the realisation that she may die soon may be added reasons for wanting to fulfil herself in some way before she dies, and to leave something of herself after she is gone; studies have shown that women with HIV infection are no more likely to have their pregnancy terminated than other women who are at risk of HIV infection but are HIV negative (e.g. Selwyn *et al.* 1988).

Women who are HIV positive need individual advice and sensitive counselling allowing them to make their own decision about pregnancy in the light of their individual medical and social situation. If a woman decides that she does want to conceive, she needs advice about how to do so while minimising the risk of infecting her partner or of becoming re-infected by him. She can learn to recognise when she is most likely to conceive and avoid intercourse or use barrier contraception at other times. This is known as 'reverse Billings': most women experience a few days or more after a menstrual period when they produce very little vaginal secretion and feel 'dry'; around the time that a woman ovulates, she will produce more mucus and will start to feel 'wet' again. This is the time that she is most likely to conceive.

A woman who discovers her HIV status during pregnancy will need support in coming to terms with such devastating news at a time when she may feel particularly vulnerable. She needs immunological and virological testing so that an assessment of the risk to her and to her baby can be made, thus enabling her to make an informed decision about the future of her pregnancy.

Transmission of HIV through breast feeding

There have been a handful of reported cases of postnatal transmission of HIV infection from an infected mother to her baby via breast milk, usually in cases where the mother acquired the infection from a blood transfusion given after birth. One study (Ziegler *et al*. 1988) suggests that the risk is greatest if the mother seroconverts while she is breast feeding, perhaps due to the presence of large numbers of HIV in the blood at that time.

As we have seen (p. 46), it is not possible to be certain whether a baby is infected until some months after birth. Although it has been suggested that breast feeding after an 'antibody positive' pregnancy may not involve any additional risk (Ziegler *et al*. 1988), it would seem sensible, in countries such as Britain and the US where safe alternatives to breast feeding are available, for HIV-infected mothers to be informed about the possible risk and discouraged from breast feeding. However, the risk of infection from breast feeding is clearly very small. A number of studies (e.g. in Zaire and Haiti) have found that breast and bottle-fed babies of HIV positive mothers did not differ in their likelihood of becoming infected with HIV (Panos Institute 1990). Thus, in countries where safe alternatives to breast feeding may not be available, the additional risk of infection from breast feeding may be less than the dangers to the baby's health of not breast feeding.

Women at high risk of infection (those still injecting drugs or partners of men with HIV infection) should be informed of the potential risks of breast feeding.

In summary, pregnancy does not seem to be dangerous for women with HIV infection as long as they remain well. Furthermore, the risk of infecting the baby may be less than was thought. On the basis of immunological and virological tests, women can be offered individual advice about the risk of pregnancy to them and to their baby. Women with HIV infection or those at high risk of infection should be informed of the potential risk of breast feeding.

HETEROSEXUAL TRANSMISSION

A woman with HIV infection will want to know how likely she is to infect her sexual partner if he is uninfected. A woman who is uninfected but whose partner is HIV positive will want to know how likely she is to become infected.

HIV infection is poorly transmitted during sexual intercourse compared to other sexually transmitted diseases such as gonorrhoea (Alexander 1990). Some people have had regular unprotected intercourse over some years with an HIV positive partner without becoming infected. Nevertheless, other people – men and women – have become infected after a single act of vaginal intercourse (e.g. Johnson 1988). It seems that some people are more infectious than others, and that some people are more susceptible to infection than others (Bury 1989). Anal intercourse is riskier for women than vaginal intercourse because the anal canal is more likely to be damaged during penetration than the vagina. However, anal intercourse is a less common sexual practice, with the result that more women overall have become infected through vaginal intercourse than anal intercourse (Johnson 1990).

A person with HIV infection may infect his or her sexual partner during vaginal or anal intercourse at any time, although they may be more likely to do so at the time of seroconversion and later on in the disease as they become ill. People with HIV infection are also more likely to infect their partner if either has genital ulceration or genital warts (Alexander 1990). There is some evidence that men with HIV infection are slightly more likely to infect their female sexual partners than women with HIV infection are to infect their male sexual partners, but there is no doubt that both can happen (Johnson and Laga 1988, Alexander 1990).

The risk of transmitting HIV infection during kissing or oral sex is very small – there have been only a handful of cases reported worldwide. Heterosexual and lesbian couples, where one is infected with HIV, may wish to reduce the risk of transmission still further by avoiding oral sex during menstruation or by using latex barriers such as dental dams (see p. 54).

Some couples may continue to have unprotected intercourse for some years without HIV being transmitted sexually to the uninfected partner. They may then find it difficult to accept the need to avoid intercourse or to use barriers to prevent infection as the disease progresses and the transmission of infection becomes more likely.

A woman who is HIV positive may have a partner who is also infected with HIV. They may assume that there is nothing to be gained by using barrier protection but there are a number of reasons why this is not the case. She may be exposed to re-infection by HIV at every act of intercourse and this may increase the risk of progression of her disease. If she did not acquire her infection from her current partner (via intercourse or sharing of needles) he may be infected by another strain of the virus which may be more virulent than her own. Unprotected sexual intercourse also puts the woman at risk of acquiring other sexually transmitted infections which could further suppress her immunity and thus increase the speed of progression of her HIV disease (Weber *et al.* 1986). Thus, unprotected intercourse continues to pose a theoretical risk for an HIV positive woman whose partner is HIV positive.

CONTRACEPTION FOR WOMEN WHO ARE HIV POSITIVE

Women who are HIV positive may want to use contraception to prevent pregnancy as well as using a barrier to protect them and their partners against infection or re-infection. Any method should not increase the risk of transmitting HIV infection nor increase the risk of progression of their HIV disease. Apart from theoretical considerations about efficacy and safety, it is essential to take into account the woman's individual circumstances and the likelihood that she will use the recommended method. In practice, the most effective method is the one she is happy to use but she also needs to know that it is safe for her health.

Many drug-using women have disrupted menstrual cycles, with long gaps between periods, and may assume that they are unlikely to conceive. Such women may find it particularly difficult to accept their need for contraception.

Protection against pregnancy

Combined oral contraception

Many drug users have liver damage due to a past history of hepatitis and this damage could be made worse by taking the combined pill. It is therefore important for drug users or ex-drug users to have their liver function checked and, if abnormal, they should not be offered the combined pill.

The combined pill, particularly the oestrogen component, has been shown to suppress the immune system (Bousquet and Fizet 1984). Injecting drugs, especially opiate drugs, is also known to suppress the immune system (Sonnex 1987). Nevertheless, there is no evidence to suggest that the use of combined oral contraception affects the progression of HIV disease (WHO 1987). Certain anxieties remain, however. The immunological suppression of pregnancy seems to be significant in HIV disease only once the woman's immune system has been severely damaged. Similarly, although oral contraception seems to be safe for women with HIV disease as long as they do not have liver damage and remain well, the immunosuppression caused by the pill may become significant once the woman's immune system shows signs of damage. This theoretical possibility will cause a dilemma as, at this stage of the disease, a woman needs the most efficient contraception to prevent pregnancy. If no other method is suitable, and in the absence of evidence to back up this theory, it may be better for a woman to continue on the pill rather than risk pregnancy. 'Pregnancy produces far more pronounced immunodeficiency than that which might result from use of any hormonal method of contraception' (WHO 1987).

Another factor to consider is that some women with HIV infection may find that their lives are too chaotic to take the pill regularly.

Progestogen-only contraception

There is no evidence that low dose progestogen pills significantly affect liver function or suppress immunity (Sonnex 1987, WHO 1987). However, the need to take this method even more regularly than the combined pill may make it unsuitable for many women.

Injectable progestogens

High dose depot progestogens, administered in the form of a three-monthly injection, have less effect on liver function and on immunity than the combined pill. This method does not require daily motivation and may therefore be acceptable to current or ex-drug users whose liver function should be monitored regularly during their use.

Intra-uterine contraceptive device (IUD) e.g. the coil

This is also an effective method of contraception that does not require continuing motivation but it is unsuitable for women with HIV infection. The presence of an IUD increases the risk of pelvic infection and, as already mentioned (p. 50), there is evidence that concomitant infection may increase the risk of progression of HIV disease (Weber *et al.* 1986). The increased discharge associated with the presence of an IUD could increase the number of HIV infected cells in the vagina and thus increase the risk of sexual transmission to her partner (WHO 1987). The risk of sexual transmission may also be increased where the presence of an IUD causes heavy periods (WHO 1987). The insertion of an IUD may be associated with slight inflammation or damage to the wall of the uterus which could facilitate virus entry (WHO 1987). Thus a woman with HIV infection or at high risk of infection should not be offered the IUD and, if an IUD is already present, it is advisable to have it removed.

Sterilisation

Some women with HIV infection may choose to be sterilised and there is no evidence that this poses any danger as long as the woman remains well. One study has suggested that surgical trauma may precipitate the development of AIDS (Konotey-Ahulu 1987) so sterilisation is perhaps best avoided in those whose immune system is already severely damaged by HIV infection, although this will need to be balanced against the greater risk of immunosuppression due to pregnancy.

Post-coital (emergency) contraception

The post-coital IUD should not be offered to women with HIV infection. There is, however, no contra-indication to the post-coital pill for women with HIV infection as there is no evidence that it suppresses immunity.

Methods that also offer a barrier to HIV transmission

Diaphragm

It is not yet known how HIV passes from male semen into the female blood-stream. If transmission is through the cervix, the diaphragm may protect the woman from re-infection but if infection is through the vaginal walls then it will not. It is also not known whether the male becomes infected by HIV in cervical mucus or in vaginal secretions; if the latter, then the diaphragm will not protect the male from infection. There is also some theoretical concern that the insertion of the diaphragm could cause slight trauma to the vagina, making passage of the virus from male to female more likely. On theoretical grounds, the diaphragm used with a spermicide containing nonoxynol–9 (see p. 53) should be effective protection for a woman against re-infection and for her male partner against infection but there is, as yet, no epidemiological or laboratory evidence to support this.

Condoms

Condoms have been shown to prevent the transmission of HIV in the laboratory, as they are impermeable to HIV (Conant *et al.* 1986, Feldblum and Fortney 1988). In practice, however, condoms may burst or leak, or they may be damaged by oil-based lubricants (White *et al.* 1988) or by suppositories, creams or gels formulated using an oily base (Committee on Safety of Medicines 1988). Thus, epidemiological studies have found that the protection against transmission afforded by condoms is not foolproof (Mann *et al.* 1986, Fischl *et al.* 1987). A study on the effectiveness of the condom in practice suggests that young people with little experience of using condoms are unlikely to use them reliably in the prevention of pregnancy (Vessey *et al.* 1988) or, presumably, as barriers against infection.

In spite of these reservations, condoms are the most effective barrier so far available. They also offer additional protection against other sexually transmitted diseases (Centers for Disease Control 1988), an important added advantage for the woman with HIV infection as well as for her partner. Some women find it difficult to persuade their partners to use condoms and may need support and advice to help them to do so (see Chapters 8 and 9).

Female condom

This new contraceptive method is a polyurethane sheath which has been shown to prevent the passage of HIV in vitro (Bounds *et al.* 1988). In theory it offers a useful alternative to the male condom, particularly as its use can be controlled directly by the woman. Other advantages are that it protects the woman more effectively than the male condom against contact with semen due to leak or spillage, and it is also less likely to be damaged by oil-based lubricants (Panos Institute 1990). It can, however, be uncomfortable to use and it will be expensive to buy, so it remains to be seen whether it will become popular in practice.

Spermicides

Nonoxynol–9, the active ingredient of most spermicides used in Britain and the US, inactivates HIV in the laboratory (Hicks *et al.* 1985, Malkovsky *et al.* 1988). When tested with condoms, either in the condom or separately in the form of a pessary, foam or sponge, it provides an additional chemical barrier to HIV infection if the condom breaks or leaks (Rietmeijer *et al.* 1988). There is, however, no evidence from outside the laboratory that it protects against transmission of HIV in practice and there are reasons to think it might not. For example, the spermicide may not mix effectively enough with the ejaculate for all the virus to be destroyed (Alexander 1990). One virologist has raised the possibility that nonoxynol–9 might even enhance the risk of infection by damaging the lining of the genital tract, by impairing local immune defences or by activating lymphocytes, the cells which are targeted by HIV (Jeffries 1988). The advisability of recommending nonoxynol–9-containing spermicides for the prevention of HIV transmission has now been questioned (Bird 1991) and recent Family Planning Association and Health Education Authority leaflets no longer recommend the use of this spermicide.

In spite of these reservations, the range of formulations of nonoxynol–9 available make these spermicides acceptable to some women who are unwilling to use any other method (Bury 1988). In practice, a woman should be advised that if she experiences any discomfort or irritation when using a spermicide, she should stop using it.

Other spermicides such as benzalkonium chloride and chlorhexidine have also been shown to destroy HIV in the laboratory and are being investigated further (Alexander 1990).

Latex barriers or dental dams

These are squares of latex that can be used to protect against the transmission of HIV infection during oral sex with a woman. There has been no published study of their effectiveness but, as they are made of the same material as condoms, they can be expected to reduce the risk of transmission if used carefully.

In summary, there is no barrier method which offers complete protection against the transmission of HIV infection. Therefore, the only way to prevent sexual transmission of the virus is to avoid penetrative intercourse. If this is not an option, a couple will need to use a barrier method and the current evidence suggests that a condom used with a spermicide probably offers the most protection. Thus, the most effective barrier depends on the co-operation of the male partner. A number of authors have commented on the lack of research on methods that women can use without the need for male co-operation (e.g. Anonymous 1990, Stein 1990).

If a woman wishes to avoid pregnancy she also needs to use a more effective contraceptive. As long as she remains well, she has a choice of an oral contraceptive, a depot (injectable) progestogen or sterilisation, but once her immune system has been severely damaged, a depot progestogen may be the safest. If she has an IUD it would be advisable to have it removed.

REFERENCES

Ades, A.E., Parker S., Berry, T., Holland, F.J., Davison, C.F., Cubitt, D., Hjelm, M., Wilcox, A.H., Hudson, C.N., Briggs, M., Tedder, R.S. and Peckham, C.S. (1991) 'Prevalance of maternal HIV infection in Thames Regions: results from anonymous published neonatal testing', *Lancet* 337: 1562-5.

Alexander, N.J. (1990) 'Sexual transmission of human immunodeficiency virus: virus entry into the male and female genital tract', *Fertility and Sterility* 54 (1): 1-18.

Anonymous (1988) 'HIV infection: obstetric and perinatal issues', *Lancet* i: 806-7.

Anonymous (1990) 'Barriers and boundaries' (editorial), *Lancet* 335: 1497-8.

Bird, K.D. (1991) 'The use of spermicide containing nonoxynol-9 in the prevention of HIV infection', *AIDS* 5: 791-6.

Bounds, W., Guillebaud, J., Stewart, L. and Steele, S. (1988) 'A female condom (Femshield™): a study of its user-acceptability', *British Journal of Family Planning* 14: 83-7.

Bousquet, J. and Fizet, D. (1984) 'Evidence of an immunosuppressor factor in the serum of women taking oral contraceptives', *Gynecologic and Obsteteric Investigation* 18: 178-82.

Bury, J.K. (1989) 'Counselling women with HIV infection about pregnancy, heterosexual transmission and contraception', *British Journal of Family Planning* 14 (4): 116-22.

Centers for Disease Control (1988) 'Condoms for prevention of sexually transmitted diseases', *Morbidity and Mortality Weekly Report* 37: 113-17.

Chiodo, F., Ricchi, E., Costigliola, P., Michelacci, L., Bovicelli, L. and Dallacasa, P. (1986) 'Vertical transmission of HTLV III', *Lancet* i: 739.

Committee on Safety of Medicines (1988) 'Vaginal and rectal medication and potential damage to condoms and contraceptive diaphragms', *Current Problems* No. 23.

Conant, M., Hardy, D., Sernatinger, J., Spicer, D. and Levy, J.A. (1986) 'Condoms prevent transmission of AIDS-associated retrovirus', *Journal of the American Medical Association* 255: 1706.

Ehrnst, A., Lindgren, S., Dictor, M., Johansson, B., Sonnerborg, A., Czajkowski, J., Sundin, G. and Bohlin, A.-B. (1991) 'HIV in pregnant women and their offspring: evidence for late transmission', *Lancet* 338: 203-7.

European Collaborative Study (1991) 'Children born to women with HIV-1 infection: natural history and risk of transmission', *Lancet* 337: 253-60.

Feldblum, P.L. and Fortney, J.A. (1988) 'Condoms, spermicides and the transmission of human immunodeficiency virus: a review of the literature', *American Journal of Public Health* 78: 52-4.

Fischl, M.A., Dickinson, G.M., Scott, G.B., Klimas, N., Fletcher, M.A. and Parks, W. (1987) 'Evaluation of heterosexual partners, children and household contacts of adults with AIDS', *Journal of the American Medical Association* 257: 640-4.

Hicks, D.R., Martin, L.S., Getchell, J.P., Heath, J.L., Francis, D.P., McDougal, J.S., Curran, J.W. and Voeller, B. (1985) 'Inactivation of HTLV-III/LAV-infected cultures of normal human lymphocytes by nonoxynol-9 in vitro', *Lancet* ii: 1422-3.

Jeffries, D.J. (1988) 'Nonoxynol-9 and HIV infection', *British Medical Journal* 296: 1798.

Johnson, A.M. (1988) 'Heterosexual transmission of human immunodeficiency virus', *British Medical Journal* 296: 1017-20.

Johnson, A.M. (1990) 'The epidemiology of HIV in the UK: sexual transmission', in *HIV and AIDS: An Assessment of Current and Future Spread in the UK*, UK Health Departments and Health Education Authority, London: HMSO.

Johnson, A.M. and Laga, M. (1988) 'Heterosexual transmission of HIV', *AIDS* 2: S49-S56.

Johnstone, F.D., MacCallum, L., Brettle, R., Inglis, J.M. and Peutherer, J.F. (1988)

'Does infection with HIV affect the outcome of pregnancy?', *British Medical Journal* 296: 467.

Konotey-Ahulu, F.I.D. (1987) 'Surgery and risk of AIDS in HIV positive patients', *Lancet* ii: 1146.

Lifson, A.R. and Rogers, M.R.(1986) 'Vertical transmission of HIV', *Lancet* ii: 337.

MacCallum, L.R., France, A.J., Jones, M.E., Steel, C.M., Burns, S.M. and Brettle, R.P. (1988) 'The effect of pregnancy on the progression of HIV infection'. Paper presented at IVth International Conference on AIDS, Stockholm, 12-16 June 1988.

Malkovsky, M., Newell, A. and Dalgliesh, A.G. (1988) 'Inactivation of HIV by nonoxynol-9', *Lancet* i: 645.

Mann, J., Quinn, T.C., Piot, P., Bosenge, N., Nzilambi, N., Kalala, M., Francis, H., Colebunders, R.L., Byers, R., Azila, P.K., Kabeya, N. and Curran, J.W. (1986) 'Condom use and HIV infection among prostitutes in Zaire', *New England Journal of Medicine* 316: 345.

Medical Research Council (1991) 'The unlinked anonymous HIV prevalance monitoring programme in England and Wales: preliminary results', *Communicable Disease Report* 1: 69-76.

Minkoff, H.L. (1987) 'Care of pregnant women infected with human immunodeficiency virus', *Journal of the American Medical Association* 258: 2714-17.

Mok, J.Y.Q., Giaquinto, C., de Rossi, A., Grosch-Worner, I., Ades, A.E. and Peckham, C.S. (1987) 'Infants born to mothers seropositive for human immunodeficiency virus', *Lancet* i: 1164-8.

Panos Institute (1990) *Triple Jeopardy: Women and AIDS*, London: Panos Publications.

Peckham, C.S. and Newell, M.L. (1990) 'HIV-1 infection in mothers and babies', *AIDS Care* 2(3): 205-11.

Rietmeijer, C.A.M., Krebs, J.W., Feorino, P.M. and Judson, F.N. (1988) 'Condoms as physical and chemical barriers against human immunodeficiency virus', *Journal of American Medical Association* 259: 1851-3.

Ryder, R.W., Nsa, W., Hassig, S.E., Behets, F., Rayfield, M. Ekungola, B., Nelson, A.N., Mulenda, U., Francis, H., Mwandagalirwa, K., Davachi, F., Rogers, M., Nzilamti, N., Greenberg, A., Mann, J., Quinn, T.C., Piot, P. and Curran, J.W. (1989) 'Perinatal transmission of the human immunodeficiency virus type 1 to infants of seropositive women in Zaire', *New England Journal of Medicine* 320: 1637-42.

Schoenbaum, E. E., Davenny, K. and Selwyn, P.A. (1988) 'The impact of pregnancy on HIV-related disease', in C. Hudson and F. Sharp (eds) *AIDS and Obstetrics and Gynaecology*, London: Royal College of Obstetricians and Gynaecologists.

Scott, G.B., Buck, B.E., Leterman, J.G., Bloom, F.L. and Parks, W.P. (1984) 'Acquired immunodeficiency syndrome in infants', *New England Journal of Medicine* 310: 76-81.

Scott, G.B., Fischl, M.A., Klimas, N., Fletcher, M.A., Dickinson, G.M., Levine, R.S. and Parks, W.P. (1985) 'Mothers of infants with the acquired immunodeficiency syndrome', *Journal of the American Medical Association* 253: 363-6.

Selwyn, P.A., Carter, R.J., Hartel, D., Schoenbaum, E.E. Robertson, V.J. and Klein, R.S. (1988) 'Elective termination of pregnancy among HIV seropositive and seronegative intravenous drug users'. Paper presented at IVth International Conference on AIDS, Stockholm, 12-16 June 1988.

Selwyn, P.A., Schoenbaum, E.E., Davenny, K., Robertson, V.J., Feingold, A.R.,

Shulman, J.F., Mayers, M.M., Klein, R.S., Friedland, G.H. and Rogers, M.F. (1989) 'Prospective study of human immunodeficiency virus infection and pregnancy outcome in intravenous drug users', *Journal of the American Medical Association* 261(9): 1288-94.

Sonnex, C. (1987) 'Contraception and the injecting opiate user', *British Journal of Family Planning* 13: 133-5.

Stein, Z.A. (1990) 'HIV prevention: the need for methods women can use', *American Journal of Public Health* 80: 460-2.

Tappin, D.M., Girdwood, R.W.A., Follett, E.A.C., Kennedy, R., Brown, A.J. and Cockburn, F. (1991) 'Prevalence of maternal HIV infection in Scotland based on unlinked anonymous testing of newborn babies', *Lancet* 337: 1565-7.

Vessey, M.P., Villard-Mackintosh, L., McPherson, K. and Yates, D. (1988) 'Factors influencing use-effectiveness of the condom', *British Journal of Family Planning* 14: 40-3.

Weber, J.N., McCreaner, A., Berrie, E., Wadsworth, J., Jeffries, D.J., Pinching, A.J. and Harris, J.R.W. (1986) 'Factors affecting seropositivity to human T cell lymphotropic virus type III (HTLV-III) or lymphadenopathy associated virus (LAV) and progression of disease in sexual partners of patients with AIDS', *Genito-urinary Medicine* 62: 177-80.

White, N., Taylor, K., Lyszkowski, A., Tullett, J. and Morris, C. (1988) 'Dangers of lubricants used with condoms', *Nature* 335: 19.

World Health Organisation (1987) Special Programme of Research, Development and Research Training in Human Reproduction and Special Programme on AIDS, *Report of a meeting on contraceptive methods and HIV infection*, Geneva: WHO.

Ziegler, J.B., Stewart, G.J., Penny, R., Stuckey, M. and Good, S. (1988) 'Breast feeding and transmission of HIV from mother to infant'. Paper presented at IVth International Conference on AIDS, Stockholm, 12-16 June 1988.

5 Pregnancy and HIV
Screening, counselling and services

Mary Hepburn

INTRODUCTION

In Scotland more than half of those infected with HIV acquired their infection through injecting drug use; approximately one-third of these are women. Of concern for the future is the rising number of people infected heterosexually, of whom two-thirds are women (see Chapter 1). The majority of those infected with HIV are young, with women on average younger than men and those infected through drug use younger than those infected through other routes (Communicable Diseases (Scotland) Unit, 1991). Injecting drug use closely correlates with socio-economic deprivation and, since heterosexual spread in Scotland also usually has its origins in injecting drug use, many of those infected have a background of other social problems. The situation in Scotland clearly demonstrates that HIV infection has relevance for everyone, even though many will be unaware that they are at risk. It also demonstrates the major implications for women, for their own health, for their children's health through the risk of vertical transmission, and consequently for their reproductive choices. In addition to coping with the possibility and actuality of HIV infection, many women will also have to deal with drug use or other problems due to socio-economic deprivation.

In my post as consultant obstetrician and gynaecologist I lead the team which provides the Glasgow Women's Reproductive Health Service for women with social problems. Due to the correlation between injecting drug use and social deprivation we care for many women who use drugs or are partners of drug users and consequently women with HIV infection. Our service is multidisciplinary, with contributions from a wide range of professionals both medical and non-medical, and all members of our team are experienced in dealing with the issues involved. Care is delivered through community-based clinics where women can receive help with all their problems at the same time. They can reach the service by any route they choose, including self-referral, at any time they choose, with or without an appointment. Two important elements of the service are screening and counselling.

SCREENING

There are various reasons why it might be considered advantageous to test an individual's HIV status and there are various screening methods (see Table 5.1) appropriate to these different situations. Anonymous, unattributable screening, where the test result cannot be linked to the person tested, is carried out to give information about a population rather than an individual. It provides information about the prevalence of infection and patterns of spread in various areas, and therefore allows more effective planning of services. It has been suggested that anonymous screening is unethical since it does not permit identification and consequently treatment of infected individuals. This is not a valid criticism provided attributable screening is also available, so that those who wish to determine their status can do so. For anonymous screening programmes to provide reliable and useful data however, screening of the target population must be as complete as possible and continued for a sufficiently long period of time to identify changes in prevalence. It is also essential that the programmes are well designed so that anonymity is guaranteed.

Screening which allows the result to be linked to the individual concerned is intended to enable appropriate medical care of that individual. This screening may be by either named testing or anonymous attributable testing where the person tested uses a false name (see Table 5.1). If screening of a particular group is sufficiently complete, such a programme will also provide epidemiological data, for example about prevalence.

Table 5.1 Types of HIV testing

Type of testing	Anonymous unattributable	Anonymous attributable	Named testing
Information recorded	NIL ± basic info. (e.g. age, sex, post code, risk behaviour if any)	False name Initials code numbers etc. ± basic info.	Real name ±basic info.
Linkage of test result to individual	NO	YES	YES
Identification of individual	NO	NO	YES

The screening for HIV antibodies of blood samples taken routinely from babies soon after birth to test for phenylketonuria (Guthrie test) (Peckham *et al.* 1990), is an example of an anonymous screening programme. Since the antibody detected will be maternal such testing will give information about the prevalence of HIV infection among women delivering live babies rather than among the babies themselves. The antenatal screening programmes in Lothian and Tayside (Goldberg *et al.* 1992) on the other hand, by using largely named screening (with the option of anonymous unattributable testing) gives information about the women concerned as well as about the population as a whole.

Where a result can be linked to the individual concerned who is to be informed of the result, it is essential that full and appropriate counselling is provided both before and after the test to ensure understanding of the issues involved and to allow informed choice. Such counselling should not be given only to those who perceive themselves to be at risk, otherwise those who feel they are not at risk may simply undergo screening with the assumption that the test will be negative rather than acknowledging the possibility that it may be positive. Counselling in this context is largely provision of information to allow informed choice – it is definitely not the giving of advice and should not be in any way directive.

WHY IDENTIFY THOSE INFECTED?

There is still considerable confusion about why it might be advantageous to try to identify those infected with HIV. The notion persists among some health care workers, as well as in the population in general, that identification and screening of individuals perceived to be at particularly high risk of acquiring HIV infection will protect those in contact with them from infection. This is illogical for a number of reasons. First, many people are not aware that they are at risk, so screening only 'high risk' individuals would be insufficient (Krasinski *et al.*, 1988, Barbacci *et al.* 1991). Even if everyone were screened however, it would not be possible to identify all those infected, for while a positive result confirms infection, a negative one does not exclude it, since it takes some time for seroconversion to occur. Moreover, if there is ongoing risky behaviour, infection may occur after testing, and even screening repeated at regular intervals could not guarantee identification of all those infected. The only logical and safe approach therefore is to assume that everyone may be infectious and a single tier approach with universal precautions should be adopted by everyone in all aspects of life. If appropriate precautions were taken by everyone with everyone in all situations where there is potential for the virus to be transmitted, whether through sexual contact or in the care of patients by health care staff, any risk would be minimised and knowledge of an individual's HIV status would become unnecessary. There is therefore never any justification for testing an individual in the interests of some other person.

There may, however, be situations where screening might be of benefit to the woman concerned. Women contemplating pregnancy or already pregnant might feel this would give them greater choice in deciding when or whether to embark on or continue with a pregnancy. They might also wish to know so that, if infected, they could arrange medical follow-up of their child(ren). This however should be a matter of individual choice and women should not be pressurised into accepting testing.

COUNSELLING

In the context of testing for HIV infection, considerable emphasis is placed on the provision of 'counselling' and the need for those providing it to possess the necessary 'counselling skills'. Less attention is paid to the precise nature and purpose of such counselling. First, recognising that all women are potentially at risk of infection, it is essential that a service providing comprehensive information about all relevant aspects of HIV should be available to *all* women and not only those volunteering a history of 'high risk' behaviour. Second, testing should also be available to all women, and those who do not want anyone else to know their HIV status should have the option of having this done without giving their real name (anonymous attributable testing). Regardless of whether they decide to undergo testing, it is necessary and valuable to offer women counselling which should include information on HIV prevention. There must also be recognition of the reasons why women might have difficulty putting such information into practice. Women need sympathetic help to develop the necessary skills to use the information, with the realistic acknowledgement that any measure aimed at reducing the level of risk by however small a degree is extremely worthwhile. Thus spermicides are less effective in preventing HIV transmission than condoms (see Chapter 4) and of course penetrative intercourse with or without a condom is still riskier than non-penetrative intercourse, but many women may be unwilling or unable to achieve total elimination of risk. Information about condoms and less effective methods such as spermicides should be given in a positive way so that women do not feel guilty for choosing a compromise solution.

Women may choose to be tested before, during or after pregnancy, or not at all, depending on circumstances and other stressful factors in their lives. There should never be any pressure put on women to undergo testing at any time, even if they indicate that they are at particularly high risk of infection. Women, when pregnant, can often be persuaded to behave in a particular way, or to undergo tests or investigations, on the grounds that this is in the interests of their unborn baby, but such an argument is unjustifiable and should not be used to persuade pregnant women to undergo testing for HIV.

In addition to general information regarding HIV infection, women also need specific information regarding the relevance of HIV infection to their health and reproductive choices. Ideally such counselling should be available to all women, or at least to those contemplating pregnancy, but it should certainly be available to all women who are already pregnant. There must be recognition that much of the relevant information is either not known or imprecisely known, with the possibility that it may ultimately prove inaccurate. The information provided is therefore only the best available at the time. Thus, it has transpired that earlier estimates of the risks of pregnancy to mother and baby were unduly pessimistic and it now appears (see Chapter 4) that there is no significant risk of acceleration of the progression of maternal HIV infection by pregnancy and no significant harmful effect of HIV infection on pregnancy outcome. The frequency with which vertical transmission results in fetal infection also appears to be lower than previously thought and the most recent figure of 13 per cent (approximately 1 in 8) published by the European Collaborative Study (1991), is much lower than for many other conditions which can be transmitted from mother to child, where the risk may be as high as 1 in 2 as, for example, in the case of Huntingdon's Chorea.

The relevance of these statistics to the childbearing woman with HIV infection is widely misunderstood. The precise level of risk should not be the basis on which women are advised for or against pregnancy – and indeed directive advice should not be given in any case. The acceptability of possible fetal infection is of much greater relevance to the mother, whose ultimate concern is not what proportion of children overall are infected but whether or not *her* child is infected. Emphasis on the level of risk may have an inappropriate effect, so that while a high level may be used to try to dissuade women from becoming pregnant, a belief that the level is low may encourage women to embark on pregnancy in the hope that their child will not be infected without giving consideration to that as a serious possibility. A woman needs to decide whether she could cope if *her* child were infected (including coping with the lengthy period, currently thought to be 18 months, before that question can be answered). Whether she can cope will also be influenced by the fact that not all women will share an equal desire to have children. Thus, some women would rather not become pregnant than accept any risk of their child being infected with HIV, while others consider having a child so important that any level of risk would be acceptable. Cultural, moral or religious factors might further influence their decision about contraception or termination, and it has become apparent with time that the experience of other women also exerts a noticeable effect. Early medical advice was extremely pessimistic about the outlook for both mother and baby. The fact that subsequent information has been increasingly hopeful has doubtless influenced women's choices but even more important is the fact that this information is demonstrably true. Increasing numbers of friends or acquaintances with HIV infection having healthy uninfected babies may persuade other women with HIV infection that pregnancy constitutes a reasonable risk and one which they too would be prepared to take.

Ultimately, the acceptability of risk is an individual matter which women must feel free to decide for themselves (or at any rate with their partners or families). Service providers should respect that freedom and refrain either from giving directive advice or from expressing their personal opinion of the woman's decision once it has been made; their role is to provide the necessary information to allow women to make an informed choice and then to provide them, in as non-judgemental a way as possible, with the help and support to implement that choice.

Of relevance for those women who choose to become pregnant, is the information that longer duration of infection may be associated with a higher risk of transmitting infection to the child (see Chapter 4). Whilst it might be reasonable to give this information so that women do not unnecessarily delay a planned pregnancy, for example in the belief that a cure is imminent, great care is needed in deciding whether, when or how to give this information as it may put women under considerable stress if their circumstances are not appropriate for a pregnancy at that time.

The next important point about counselling women with HIV infection is that it must include planning and help with the practical issues. Women need to consider whom they would choose to tell about their HIV status and possible responses of family, friends, professionals and members of the public with whom they come in contact. They need information about problems they may encounter regarding their child's health as well as their own, the family's social and financial situation, and where they can obtain help. They also need to consider possible difficulties that might arise from their child's social contact with others, either inside or outside the home; while there is a negligible risk to others from social contact with the child (although the reverse may be true in that the child who is immunocompromised as a result of HIV infection will be more susceptible to infection and consequently more at risk from other children) there may be a mistaken perception of great risk, resulting in prejudice and discrimination.

It is important to realise that the various aspects of HIV infection described cannot be covered in one session and, indeed, any attempt to do so might mean that much of the information might not be retained. This is particularly true when giving information to women who have just discovered they are

HIV positive. The process is an ongoing one, which women must have the opportunity to work through gradually, involving partners, family or friends at various times if they so wish, with access preferably to the same counsellor each time, but certainly to a small number of professionals.

The final important point about HIV counselling is that the problem of HIV infection should be viewed not in isolation but always in the context of associated or predisposing problems. For example, while not all women with or at risk of HIV infection use drugs, drug-related problems will be important to a great number, either because of their own use or use by their partner, a relative or friend.

DRUGS IN PREGNANCY

Pregnant women feel a great sense of responsibility for their unborn child and pregnancy can provide a great stimulus for behavioural change. This is no less true for women who use drugs, who are usually very concerned about the health of their child and often highly motivated to stop using drugs during pregnancy. Unfortunately, current opinion on management of drug use in pregnancy includes a number of conflicting and incompatible views. Thus, while drug use by pregnant women is regarded as harmful to the unborn baby, causing increased rates of mortality and morbidity, detoxification in pregnancy is allegedly even more harmful to the fetus (Rementeria and Nunag 1973, Perlmutter 1974, Fraser 1976, Vaille 1985). Furthermore, it could be argued that detoxification is often unsuccessful, leading to continued injection of illicit drugs and consequently continued exposure to the risk of HIV infection. The standard advice is therefore that maintenance substitution therapy should be prescribed at a constant level throughout the pregnancy. After delivery however, abstinence has often been regarded as essential for adequate child care and considerable pressure is sometimes put on women to become drug free immediately, at a time when they are under a great deal of stress.

Our experience in caring for more than 200 women using drugs during pregnancy suggests that this approach is neither correct nor helpful. First, it has not been our experience that detoxification during pregnancy is unduly harmful to the baby and in fact we have not observed any adverse effects whatsoever as a consequence of maternal detoxification at any stage of pregnancy. Equally, it has not been our experience that continued use, or at least continued opiate use, causes major long-term harm to the baby. Continued use may result in withdrawal symptoms in the newborn baby, and although the level of drug use by the mother during pregnancy does not correlate exactly with the severity of withdrawal symptoms in the baby, in general the greater the level of use, the more serious the baby's illness and there is no doubt that some babies can be very ill indeed. These neonatal withdrawal symptoms are also extremely distressing to the mother and may necessitate the baby's admission to the Special Care Nursery and, hence, its separation from the mother. Any attempt to control the level of the mother's drug use antenatally is therefore of value and in our service has resulted in a very low incidence of withdrawal symptoms and an even lower incidence of symptoms requiring treatment. This is, however, a short-term problem. The adverse pregnancy outcomes (including a higher incidence of perinatal death and of premature and low birthweight babies) reported elsewhere (Perlmutter 1974, Connaughton *et al.* 1977, Bolton 1987) have not been observed among women under our care and may simply reflect the general effects of socio-economic deprivation, which correlates closely with drug use. The concentration by our service on addressing social problems and trying to promote stability of lifestyle with consequent earlier and more regular attendance for health care and reduction of stress may go some way towards explaining the more favourable pregnancy outcomes experienced by women attending our service.

Second, while detoxification may indeed be unsuccessful, with continued injection of drugs, maintenance therapy is equally no guarantee against continued injection and the risk of HIV infection should be regarded as a separate issue. Even if abstinence proves short lived, it is still worthwhile and detoxification repeated at intervals throughout pregnancy may promote greater overall stability of drug use. Thus, in my view women should be allowed to attempt detoxification during pregnancy if they wish but there should also be the option of maintenance therapy for those who cannot or do not want to attempt detoxification.

Finally, the view that maternal drug use is incompatible with adequate child care is unjustified. Of greater importance than the drug use per se, is its effect on lifestyle; thus, the woman whose drug use is under control may be a very adequate mother and management should be directed towards offering help and support to maintain that stability rather than adopting a confrontational approach which demands proof of her drug-free status.

It would therefore appear that neither detoxification nor continued drug use during or after pregnancy has as great a direct effect as previously thought. The major impact of drug use both on pregnancy and child care would appear to result from the indirect effects of deprivation and multiple social problems, either predisposing to or as a consequence of drug use. Consequently, no woman should ever lose custody of her child simply because she uses drugs; it would be more appropriate to regard drug use as yet another one of the wide range of social problems requiring the availability of a range of services. There should also be much earlier involvement of social services in a role concerned more with support and prevention than with crisis intervention, and with the objective of enabling children wherever possible to remain in the custody of their mothers. The problems of drug use and consequently of HIV infection can only be adequately dealt with if all the underlying problems are addressed.

DELIVERY OF SERVICES

If women are to receive effective help with HIV-related problems, there must be provision of effective and appropriate services which women are both able and happy to use. Unfortunately, current services often fail to attract women and this is particularly true of services dealing with drug-related problems. This is also a reflection of the lower level of use of health care services in areas with high levels of deprivation and social problems in general. While the perception of drug services as largely directed at men may partly explain their poor level of use by women, the same explanation cannot be given for health services provided specifically for women. There are, however, a variety of reasons why women fail to attend these services.

First, there is the still widely held view that HIV affects only people who are in some way 'bad' or whose behaviour or lifestyle is unacceptable; attendance at services dealing with HIV or a request for information or screening therefore implies an admission of this type of lifestyle. There must therefore be a recognition that many women suffer shame, and fear the stigma of HIV. They also suffer the anxiety, sadly sometimes justified, that their negative views will be shared by staff and reflected in their attitudes and behaviour. Even if this is not the case, women often feel services are unlikely to provide them with effective practical help with underlying problems. Where drug problems are involved, many women are concerned that admitting to drug use may be seen as an indicator of poor child care, of either existing children or of future children if the woman is pregnant; they fear such an admission may be used as justification for depriving them of custody of their children. Again, sadly this fear has sometimes proved to be not without foundation. A further concern about admitting drug use is that this may lead to pressure to accept HIV testing, with the further fear that a positive test may result in pressure not to embark on or continue with a pregnancy – yet again, a fear with a basis in fact!

Apart from concerns about possible treatment, women with other social problems often simply do not have time to attend services; dealing with problems relating to housing, financial or legal difficulties may have much greater immediacy for them and it is observed time and again that women place the needs and health of their families before their own health interests. The woman who is infected with HIV has an even greater problem: the many additional services she is required to attend may be very time-consuming, leaving her with no chance of a normal life. Not only does attending services occupy much of her time but it ensures that the problems of HIV remain firmly in the forefront of her mind, which can prove to be very stressful. In addition, attendance at or the need to attend so many services may result in women suffering a real and perceived loss of control over their lives. It is therefore desirable to co-ordinate services to make them as efficient and unobtrusive as possible. We have found that organisation of services on a multidisciplinary basis is even better and if women can obtain help with all their social, economic and legal problems at the same place as they receive health care, it makes life much easier for them. Access to such services should always be flexible and easy so that women can get help with problems very quickly as they arise. For example in our service, while clinics obviously cannot operate 24 hours a day, 7 days a week, they do when open allow access without a fixed appointment or without a formal referral. Our six clinics operate in different areas on different days and if women need help on a day their regular or nearest clinic is not open they can attend whichever clinic (if any) is operating at the time; in times of major crisis when immediate help is required, whether outside clinic hours or not, they can contact or attend the in-patient ward in the maternity hospital which is staffed at all times by team members familiar with their problems.

Therefore, if women infected or affected by HIV are to be encouraged to use services, it is important that services should be developed to meet their needs and wishes. This cannot be done without consulting the women themselves. Services should be easy and pleasant to use, efficiently organised and integrated to provide help with as many issues as possible at a single site, thus removing the time consuming need to attend large numbers of single services. Staff attitudes should be sympathetic, non-judgemental and supportive. Women should be involved in design and delivery of services on an ongoing basis and also involved in deciding the details of their own personal care. They should be encouraged to exercise choice without the fear that they will be seen as irresponsible or unco-operative if they choose not to accept a particular service. As discussed, service providers must be careful not to impose their own views on women and should try to help the women retain as much control over their lives as possible. If services fail to attract women, it is difficult to offer the help they need, but if women choose not to attend it must be acknowledged that the problem may lie with the services rather than with the women; services are, after all, intended to improve the quality of life not detract from it.

REFERENCES

Barbacci, M., Repke, J.T., Chaisson, R.E. (1991) 'Routine prenatal screening for HIV infection', *Lancet* 337: 709–11.

Bolton, P.J. (1987) 'Drugs and abuse', in D.F. Hawkins (ed.) *Drugs in Pregnancy: Human Teratogenesis and Related Problems*, p. 180–210. London: Churchill Livingstone.

Communicable Diseases (Scotland) Unit (1991) 'Human immunodeficiency virus type 1 (HIV+) antibody report to 30 June 1991', *Answer* (AIDS News Supplement, CDS Weekly Report) 91/29.

Connaughton, J.F., Reeser, D., Schut, J. and Finnegan, L.P. (1977) 'Perinatal addiction: outcome and management', *American Journal of Obstetrics and Gynaecology* 129: 679–86.

European Collaborative Study (1991) 'Children born to women with HIV-1 infection: natural history and risk of transmission', *Lancet* 337: 253–60.

Fraser, A.C. (1976) 'Drug addiction in pregnancy', *Lancet* ii: 896–9.

Goldberg, D.J., MacKinnon, H., Smith, R., Patel, N.B., Scrimegour, J.B., Inglis, J.M., Peutherer, J.F., Urquhart, G.E., Emslie, J.A.N., Covell, R.G. and Reid, D. (1992) 'Prevalence of HIV among childbearing women having termination of pregnancy: multi-disciplinary steering group study', *British Medical Journal* 304: 1082–85.

Johnstone, F.D. (1990) 'Drug abuse in pregnancy', *Contemporary Review of Obstetrics and Gynaecology* 2: 96–103.

Krasinski, K., Borrowsky, W., Bebenroth, D. and Moore, T. (1988) 'Failure of voluntary testing for human immunodeficiency virus to identify infected parturient women in a high risk population' (correspondence) *New England Journal of Medicine* 318: 185.

Peckham, C.S., Tedder, R.S., Briggs, M., Ades, A.E., Hjelm, M., Wilcox, A.H., Parra-Mejia, N. and O'Connor, C. (1990). 'Prevalence of maternal HIV infection based on unlinked anonymous testing of newborn babies', *Lancet* 335: 516-19.

Perlmutter, J. (1974) 'Heroin addiction and pregnancy', *Obstetrical and Gynaecological Survey* 29: 439–46.

Rementeria, J.L. and Nunag, N.N. (1973) 'Narcotic withdrawal in pregnancy. Stillbirth incidence with a case report', *American Journal of Obstetrics and Gynaecology* 116: 1152–6.

Vaille, C. (1985) 'Risks incurred by children of drug-addicted women: some medical and legal aspects', *Bulletin on Narcotics* 37: 149–56.

Part III
Prostitution

6 HIV and the sex industry

Ruth Morgan Thomas

Throughout this chapter I will be using certain terms with which readers may not be familiar and which perhaps require some clarification:

> *Sex industry* – when the term 'prostitution' is used people focus on the prostitute as though prostitution were something that prostitutes do on their own and amongst themselves. Consumers, managers, police and other controllers of the sex industry are too often forgotten or ignored. Prostitution is a business which operates under commercial market forces; the work element and the impact that others have on the working conditions in the sex industry are often neglected.
> *Sex worker* is used to define those, both male and female, who accept some form of payment in return for physical sexual services. The term 'prostitute' often invokes a stereotypical image of a 'street woman' or 'high class call girl' and ignores the enormous range of people providing commercial sex. This paper addresses issues common to both male and female sex workers but focuses primarily on issues facing *women* as sex workers.

UNDERLYING ATTITUDES TO THE SEX INDUSTRY AND SEX WORKERS

It is time to move away from the concept of 'high risk groups', such as prostitutes, intravenous drug users and homosexuals. The fact that a person accepts money for sexual services or injects drugs or has sex with someone of the same gender does not in itself put them at risk of HIV infection. It is how people engage in specific high risk activities that can put them at risk.

HIV is sexually transmitted and since sex is an integral part of the sex industry, it is not surprising that HIV and AIDS are being linked with the sex industry. What is dubious, however, is the way in which this link is being interpreted not only by the tabloid press but even by a few experts in the field.

The assumption seems to be that the inclusion of some form of payment somehow transforms any commercial sexual act into a high risk activity, regardless of risk reduction strategies employed or the HIV status of those involved.

'Prostitutes spread AIDS' seems to be a statement accepted without question or thought, whereas 'Prostitutes prevent AIDS' is an unacceptable or challenging concept for many. It is the first of these statements which appears to underlie many people's attitude to sex work and to influence the slant of many research projects examining the issues around HIV and the sex industry. The most disturbing aspect of this is that the focus has been directed at sex workers with the underlying assumption that most, if not all, sex workers have AIDS, and if they have not already got 'IT', that they are not interested in preventing themselves from becoming infected. Attention and fear have centred around female sex workers infecting 'members of the general public', that is, 'normal' heterosexual males and thereby their 'normal' heterosexual partners. It would appear that clients bear no responsibility for their actions and are merely victims of the 'evil and predatory' sex workers. Yet no sex worker forces a client to have sex, protected or unprotected, whereas threats of, or actual, physical violence including rape, in order to obtain unprotected penetrative sex are a far from rare experience, especially for women working the streets. The buck apparently stops with the sex worker, as being the person ultimately responsible for infecting 'decent' people, regardless of the source of her own infection. Those who are already seropositive did not set out with the intention of becoming infected, nor are they setting out with the intention of infecting others. Are we really interested in ascribing guilt to individuals or groups?

No-one, least of all sex workers, denies that there is a risk of transmission of HIV in commercial penetrative sexual contacts, just as there is in any penetrative sexual contact outside a lifelong monogamous relationship. However, no-one would advocate celibacy across the board, nor is it realistic to expect that everyone will have only one sexual partner for their entire life. It is accepted that it is possible to reduce the risk of sexual transmission of HIV by using condoms and by other risk reduction strategies. This applies equally to both commercial and non-commercial sex.

HISTORICAL CONTEXT OF SEX WORK AND PROPHYLAXIS IN THE SEX INDUSTRY

Sex work is one of the oldest professions known and the many attempts to eradicate the sex industry have failed throughout history. There have always been those who are prepared to pay for sexual services, just as there have always been those prepared to provide them, despite the many restrictions and laws attempting to regulate sex workers and their clients and despite many threats to the well-being, health or lives of sex workers and clients.

Sex workers have long been stigmatised; their profession often excludes them from society which regards itself as 'respectable', 'decent' or 'normal'.

Any woman suspected of such behaviour is likely to acquire the social status of 'prostitute'. That status makes her vulnerable to legal controls and punishment and brands her the prototype 'whore'... a heavily stigmatised social status which in most societies remains fixed regardless of change in behaviour. Often women who themselves view sex work as temporary and part-time work, are forced by legal and social labelling to remain prostitutes and to bear the prostitute status in all aspects of their lives.

(Pheterson 1990: 398–9)

For these very reasons sex workers have often responded to the 'whore stigma' by leading double lives and hiding their involvement in the sex industry from family, friends and acquaintances. In addition women tend not to divulge their working lives to statutory and voluntary agencies for fear of repercussions. Women with children are too often assumed to be unfit parents if they are, or ever have been, involved in the sex industry. Their ability to raise their children 'properly' is questioned and many fear that their children may be taken into care if they are discovered. Few sex workers will list their sex work experience on their curriculum vitae for fear that it would destroy their chance of employment. This adds to the economic problems faced by women seeking alternative employment, as they have to explain why there are gaps in their employment history. While sex work is stigmatised, the 'whore stigma' will continue to make women involved in sex work vulnerable and lacking any power to change their standing in society.

Involvement in the sex industry has always been associated with the possibility of physical violence, but sex workers have no control over the number of attacks targeted at them. Nor is their situation helped by police reactions when sex workers report criminal acts of physical violence and rape. They are often told that it is only to be expected if they are involved in sex work. Society, through our police forces, seems to be saying that such attacks are to some extent justified and that sex workers have no right to the protection of the law.

HIV infection is not the first possibly fatal or incurable sexually transmitted disease; the cure for syphilis has only been found in the last fifty years. Those involved in the sex industry have acknowledged throughout history the threat posed to them by sexually transmitted diseases. The prophylactic benefits, for which they were originally designed, and subsequently the contraceptive benefits of condoms have long been recognised by female sex workers. Condoms, made from linen or animal membrane were available, at a price, in London by 1666 (Parisot 1987). While sexually transmitted diseases continued to prevail and no cure was available, prophylaxis was seen as the only alternative and the use of condoms by sex workers can be found in writings and art from the seventeenth century onwards. In the twentieth century, with the arrival of cures for most sexually transmitted diseases and the discovery of the female contraceptive pill, the condom has fallen from popularity, despite advances in both comfort and efficacy. However, many female sex workers have continued to regard the prevention of sexually transmitted diseases and the desire for a barrier between themselves and their clients as a priority. Various means of prophylaxis are currently used by sex workers around the world – condoms, spermicides, regular prophylactic courses of antibiotics, douching, herbal remedies and, in some cultures, talismans. Not all provide adequate protection but they do show a degree of awareness.

Social scientists have long sought a possible explanation for why women enter sex work and many have attempted to define psychological and social characteristics of such women (Benjamin and Masters 1964, Bullough and Bullough 1978). Again the focus has been on sex workers, rather than on their clients who vastly outnumber them. In Europe as many as one in six men are believed to be clients of sex workers (B. Obriste, personal communication). A model of 'susceptibility' has been developed in which it is argued that criteria such as 'a feeling of complete worthlessness' (Bess and Janus 1976), 'alienation' (Brown 1979) and 'self-abasement' (Bullough 1965) predispose certain women to enter sex work. Personal crisis (Maerov 1965) and traumatic events such as incest or rape (James 1976) have all been identified as part of this susceptibility model. Alongside this concept of susceptibility comes the concept of exposure (Bryan 1965, Davis 1971, Hirschi 1972) where contact with those already involved in the sex industry, and sufficient inducements, again predispose certain women. Support for this theory has come from case histories of women involved in the sex industry (e.g. Greenwald 1958). However, none of these studies included control groups of women from similar backgrounds who had never engaged in sex work, nor did their samples represent a cross section of those involved in sex work. In those few studies that have included a control group, no distinct differences between the psychological or social characteristics of sex workers and non-sex workers could be defined (Gray 1973, Polonsky 1974, Exner *et al.* 1977, Potterat *et al.* 1985).

The reason most sex workers would give for their involvement in the sex industry is that it provides them with the best, or in some cases their only, option for supporting themselves and their dependents. It enables them to maintain a standard of living which is not available through the state welfare system and in some cases provides the financial foundation for future security. Money, or rather the lack of it, is a powerful motive in seeking any form of employment. Sex work is the means by which some people choose to earn their living or subsidise whatever other income they may have to meet their needs.

THE SEX INDUSTRY AS PUBLIC HEALTH THREAT – PAST AND PRESENT

The sex industry, or more specifically the sex worker, has long been perceived as a public health threat. Military leaders throughout history have been concerned about the levels and effects of sexually transmitted diseases amongst their troops, particularly during wartime. Sex workers were seen as a major threat, as is clearly illustrated by much of the health education propaganda (e.g. 'A German bullet is cleaner than a whore') issued during World War II. Darrow (1984) has pointed out that '... the recognition of prostitution as a social problem (i.e. civilian as well as military) emerged in the middle of the nineteenth century'. From this point onwards there has been experimentation with ways of controlling sex work and thereby supposedly controlling the health threat.

Four basic solutions to the perceived social problems created by the sex industry have been tried:

1 *Regimentation* which requires sex workers to be registered and licensed by the police or state, to reside in and restrict their sexual activities to segregated areas, to be inspected regularly for sexually transmitted diseases and to be quarantined 'until cured' when found to be infected.
2 *Abolition* which aimed at emancipating society from all 'social evils' and eradicating the sex industry.
3 *Prohibition* which attempted to combine both the previous strategies by officially suppressing the sex industry while unoffically inspecting sex workers and their clients for sexually transmitted diseases.
4 *Toleration*, the best way to describe the present approach to the sex industry, emerged out of the failure of all the other strategies and in part out of the discovery of cures for gonorrhoea and syphilis. This strategy in no way condones the sex industry, as it involves periodic and often symbolic repression of sex workers. Legal restrictions on the way the sex industry operates were introduced, aimed at reducing the 'nuisance' and 'exploitation' of sex workers. None of this legislation has given any thought to enabling sex workers to minimise health risks at work: most of the enforcement of the law is directed at sex workers, and has often led to

them becoming more vulnerable both to clients and to those who control the sex industry.

All these strategies have attempted in some way to regulate or eradicate the sex industry; all have failed. In addition, they have failed to improve the situation of the sex worker with regard to preventing the transmission of sexually transmitted diseases within commercial sexual contacts, and in many cases have made it worse. The sex industry exists, every society has its own variation, and we must learn how to live with it. The primary aim should be to control sexually transmitted diseases including HIV infection and not to control sex workers.

THE SEX INDUSTRY TODAY

Sex work, that is the exchange of physical sexual services for payment, is not illegal in Britain, although it is in some other countries. However, soliciting, procuring, pandering, running a brothel (an establishment having more than one sex worker on duty) and living off the earnings of a sex worker are all illegal under British civil or criminal law. The result of this is that it is almost impossible to engage in sex work without some law being broken by sex workers, their partners/dependents, their clients or those running the sex industry. A variety of working situations and strategies have developed in an attempt to meet the demands of clients while minimising the opportunity for physical violence and the repercussions of the law for those involved in the sex industry.

The most visible and often the most vulnerable women are those who work on the streets, often working in dark and isolated locations which offer no protection from attack and harassment. Some women will choose to work from bars or clubs which allows them more time to negotiate with clients. This is particularly so when police crack down on street work or when attacks on women escalate. Both street and bar workers are independent and, apart from occasional backhanders or 'favours' to 'important' people, they keep their earnings. They can set their own working hours, but they have little back-up if a client turns violent. Women working in fixed establishments have the protection of working indoors but have to pay a fee to the management for working. There are set hours, sometimes up to 12-hour shifts, as well as 'house rules', and in addition women may be asked to provide favours for 'important' people. Women working for 'call girl' agencies also have to pay the agency for each booking they receive as well as abiding by 'agency rules', but they are on call rather than having to work in an establishment. These women often have to pay backhanders or provide favours and they also have little back-up if clients turn violent. Women involved in sex work are a mobile population both geographically and within the various sectors of the sex industry. The needs and resources of the individual sex worker will often determine which sector of the industry she works in at that particular time, and thereby her degree of susceptibility to the demands and desires of others, while her continuing needs will determine the level of that involvement. One therefore finds women who work only occasionally when faced with financial crisis (large bills, Christmas, children's clothes, etc.), some of whom will not consider it work, through to those who consider sex work as their full-time occupation. In addition, there has been a recent trend for some women, who require considerable sums of money on a regular basis to finance their own and often their partner's drug use, to enter sex work as a means of finding the money. Others, but by no means all, who are already involved in sex work find themselves drawn into the drug culture, particularly since the sex industry has been marginalised and driven underground alongside the drug culture.

SEX WORKERS AND HIV INFECTION

The advent of HIV and the acknowledgement that it is a hetero-as well as homo-sexually transmissible disease has resulted in a large number of research projects being set up to examine levels of HIV infection amongst female sex workers. Serological testing in these studies have found levels of HIV infection amongst female sex workers to vary enormously around the world, from study group to study group, city to city, state to state and country to country.

In sub-Saharan Africa and the Caribbean Islands where seroprevalence levels are generally assumed to be high, they range from 0–88 per cent. Three out of twenty-three studies reported no evidence of HIV infection, however only two of the studies reported levels above 50 per cent. In nineteen studies carried out in Northern Africa, Asia and the Western Pacific seroprevalence ranged from 0–44 per cent. Eight studies reported no evidence of HIV infection, while two of the studies reported levels above 20 per cent. These studies show a rapid rise in the seroprevalence amongst sex workers in Thailand and India. No evidence of HIV infection has been found in a study of sex workers in Australia. In South America seroprevalence ranged from 0–9 per cent amongst studies which did not separately identify injecting drug users, with one study of injecting drug users reporting 19 per cent seroprevalence. Six out of the eleven studies reported no evidence of HIV infection. In North America, the Centers for Disease Control found seroprevalence levels ranging from 0–19 per cent amongst non-injecting drug users, with five out of eight studies reporting no evidence of HIV infection. Amongst those who reported injecting drug use, seroprevalence ranged from 0–58 per cent, with one of the eight studies finding no evidence of HIV infection. A further four studies have been carried out in North America where injecting drug users were not separately identified and seroprevalence ranged from 0–2 per cent. Five out of thirteen studies in Europe found no evidence of HIV infection; seroprevalence ranged from 0–78 per cent. Four of these studies examined injecting drug users and when they are excluded, seroprevalence levels ranged from 0–3 per cent, while amongst the studies in Spain, Italy and Switzerland, which separately identified injecting drug users, levels ranged from 48–78 per cent (Darrow 1990).

Care must be taken in extrapolating these results beyond the study groups involved because of the inherent problems of obtaining a truly representative sample of sex workers. However, some general conclusions can be drawn. It is apparent in Africa and other developing areas that transmission is primarily a result of heterosexual exposure and other co-factors unrelated to injecting drug use. The rapid rise in some areas where 'sex tourism' is promoted would suggest that the virus may be spread by 'sex tourists'. In Europe and America at present, high levels of seroprevalence are linked to the sharing of equipment amongst injecting drug users. That is not to say that heterosexual transmission is not taking place. Of the women who tested positive for HIV antibodies in the aforementioned studies, a fifth of the women in the United States, a third of the women in England, half the women in Germany and all of the women in Greece had no personal history of injecting drug use.

Seroprevalence data on clients of sex workers is extremely limited. There are cases where contact with sex workers has been listed as a risk factor. However,

> if prostitutes were effectively transmitting the virus to their customers, there would be far more cases of white heterosexual males diagnosed with AIDS than is reflected in the current statistics, because some intravenous drug users in New York have been infected with the AIDS virus since at least 1976, and a third to half of street prostitutes use intravenous drugs... However, only approximately seventy men have been diagnosed with AIDS who claim contact with prostitutes as their only risk factor, again indicating that prostitutes are not passing the disease as quickly as is commonly believed.
>
> (Alexander 1988)

Although this is based on data from the United States, a parallel could be drawn for Europe where clients of sex workers do not constitute a significant number of those with HIV infection.

PROSTITUTES PREVENT AIDS

The risk of heterosexual transmission from male to female and from female to male is real and is happening. One possible explanation for the apparent low levels of HIV transmission within commercial sex is that sex workers around the world report a willingness to use condoms and other prophylactics at work. The first International Workshop on Preventing the Sexual Transmission of HIV and Other Sexually Transmitted Diseases reported

> In our collective experience prostitutes are willing to take the responsibility for having safer sex very seriously when given the opportunity to do so. Generally speaking clients, managers and even many governments lack the same degree of commitment that we have seen amongst sex industry workers that we have worked with.
>
> (Darrow 1989)

Much has been made of the fact that some sex workers are willing to engage in unprotected penetrative sex for more money. The sex industry is a commercial business which operates under market forces. In Birmingham and Edinburgh, where research has been undertaken with clients of sex workers, both studies found approximately one-third of clients actively sought unprotected penetration (Morgan Thomas *et al.* 1990a, H Kinnell, personal communication 1990). It is necessary to examine what degree of choice the sex worker has. Is it really greed on the part of the sex worker as depicted by many people, or are there other external factors at play? When a drug addicted sex worker is offered more money – or 'double or nothing' – for unsafe sex, where is her choice if she needs her next 'fix'? When a women has to pay the management for each client she receives, regardless of whether she receives any money, where is her choice? The choice is that of the client who is demanding unprotected sex. Sex workers themselves have limited control over their working conditions; they are disempowered and vulnerable to the demands of others involved in the sex industry. If we are seeking a solution to this problem, we must not focus solely on sex workers who can do little to change their situation, but must work towards empowering them so that they cannot be exploited in this way by clients or management. It is important to emphasise that, in spite of all these pressures, there are very few sex workers, including those who have already beeen infected with HIV, who would put themselves at risk simply for a few extra pounds.

Concern has also been expressed that sex workers do not practise safe sex with their non-paying partners (Morgan Thomas *et al.* 1990b). Many women feel able to ask clients to use condoms and wish to maintain that barrier between themselves and their clients. However, they are often unable to do so in their loving relationships and have the same difficulties that any of us face in introducing condoms in our personal lives. This problem is not specific to sex workers.

Groups such as COYOTE (Call Off Your Old Tired Ethics) and the Prostitutes Collectives in Australia were set up in the late 1970s and early 1980s prior to the advent of AIDS to advocate for sex worker rights. Both groups involved the active participation of sex workers and those committed to sex worker rights and had grassroot contacts amongst both injecting and non injecting drug-using sex workers. Sex worker rights groups immediately took on board the implications of an incurable and possibly fatal sexually transmitted disease for sex workers and started HIV/AIDS education and prevention services.

Alongside the realisation that HIV can be transmitted heterosexually, female sex workers became a focus of attention for prevention work. Money suddenly became available for work with this 'high risk group' and their needs as workers and as individuals began to be addressed by those outside the sex worker rights movements. Statutory and voluntary agencies have become involved in setting up projects working with sex workers. Such agencies include: Scot-PEP (Scottish Prostitutes Education Project) and the Centenary Project in Edinburgh, Drop-In centre in Glasgow (see Chapter 7), CLASH and the Praed Street Project in London, Maryland Centre in Liverpool, Huiskammer projects in the Netherlands, sex worker projects suported by the Swiss and German AIDS Hilfe, Empower in Thailand, Talikala in the Philippines, Percago in Brazil and CAL-PEP in San Francisco. Not all these projects share a common philosophy. Some are run by Christian organisations while others are run by sex workers themselves; some are part of a statutory agency while others are independent voluntary organisations; others are research-based but also act as service providers. Some were designed to protect the sex workers while others were primarily set up to protect the clients of infected sex workers. Some projects would wish to persuade sex workers to leave the sex industry, while others have no hidden agenda and accept the sex worker's right to make her living as she chooses. However, they all share a common objective – to minimise the risks of HIV transmission within the sex industry.

A variety of services are offered to sex workers through these projects, some of which are directly related to HIV prevention; others may seem unrelated at first but are often equally important. They include: information on HIV/AIDS and transmission of the virus; provision of a range of condoms and prophylactics to cover all sexual services and client groups; health services including screening and treatment when necessary for sexually transmitted diseases, as well as primary health and dental care; drug-related services including the provision of sterile injecting equipment, education and materials for cleaning equipment, information on safer drug use, access to drug treatment programmes including maintenance on the drug of choice, medical treatment for drug-related problems, crisis support; welfare and legal services providing information and access to services; support through individual and group counselling; support in providing facilities for sex workers to meet and discuss issues; advocacy for sex workers.

None of these projects report any reticence on the part of sex workers, once informed, to comply whenever and wherever possible with safer working guidelines. All of these projects report that sex workers are still being asked for unsafe sex by clients and in some cases are being pressurised by management to comply with clients' requests.

Clearly sex workers can prevent HIV transmission within commercial sex if they are empowered to do so.

A PRAGMATIC APPROACH

Denis Altman, speaking at the first National Sex Industry Conference in Australia, stated

> we have actually stressed throughout the epidemic and throughout the safe sex behaviour programme that safe sex does not mean an end to eroticism, an end to sexual adventure, an end to sexual enjoyment. And that those things are important and essential...

> (Altman 1988)

We must not be led into using HIV/AIDS as the excuse to pass judgement on people's sexual preferences or behaviour on moral grounds. HIV/AIDS and the threat to public health has brought our attention to many 'social problems' which society has tended to ignore. It is forcing us to re-examine our attitudes and re-evaluate past and present strategies. We must take on board past experiences if we are to uncover the pitfalls that may face us in developing new and effective strategies for tackling HIV.

Public health has never been enhanced by attempts to eradicate the sex industry. Previous attempts have only served to drive commercial sex underground, where it has developed new strategies to provide for the continuing demands of clients. Nor has the criminalisation of the sex industry had any impact on curbing sex work yet its repercussions on the working conditions within the sex industry have been immense. Throughout preceding periods of prohibition and toleration, condoms have been used as evidence of illegal activities. As a result of this, sex workers on the streets have had condoms confiscated and used as evidence against them, while sex workers employed by others have had to face management resistance to promoting condom use, as condoms can still be used as evidence of brothel keeping. It is important to remember that it is the management who face prosecution for brothel keeping, not the sex workers, yet it is the women's health and lives that are at risk when condoms are not used. Criminalisation has resulted in further disempowering women with regard to their control over their working conditions, including condom use. It has also resulted in the marginalisation of sex workers so that they feel unable to take recourse to the law when attacked or robbed. As stated by Bill Darrow 'anything that drives prostitution underground obstructs, inhibits and interferes with our attempt to promote safer sex and bring about healthy behaviour changes' (Darrow 1984).

Legalising prostitution through regimentation (see p. 75), as is sometimes suggested in the interests of public health, also presents problems. Women working in Germany under such a system report difficulties in persuading clients to use condoms because the client argues that the sex worker has been given a clean bill of health by the state and he does not regard *himself* as the risk. There is the additional problem that this system also creates an illegal market of sex workers not allowed to register, such as illegal immigrants, injecting drug users and HIV positive sex workers who need to continue working. These women are already the most vulnerable and find it more problematic to come forward to health and welfare services. Further marginalising them would only increase their vulnerability to client demands.

Our aim must be to empower sex workers to take control over their working conditions, including all aspects of health and safety. At a World Health Organisation meeting on HIV and prostitution it was stated that

> Decriminalisation, i.e. the abolition (or suspension) of all laws against prostitution accompanied by a change in public opinion could diminish the marginalised position of prostitutes and in the long run improve the working conditions of voluntary prostitution by controlling them through normal business regulations... a pragmatic approach will pay off when one is concerned with sexually transmitted diseases and AIDS.
>
> (Visser 1989)

Decriminalising sex work would have an immediate impact on the working conditions of all sex workers. In particular this would allow sex workers to promote, openly and without fear of repercussions, condom use and safer sex with clients.

Drug-addicted sex workers pose different challenges with regard to HIV/AIDS prevention. If we are going to reduce their vulnerability to clients' demands then we must deal with the causes of that vulnerability. Different approaches to maintenance and/or reduction prescribing are being adopted. In some areas neither are available to drug-addicted sex workers leaving them to finance their drug use through sex work and, therefore, more vulnerable to client demands for unsafe sex. In other areas programmes, often punitive, prescribe low levels of maintenance drugs, primarily on a reduction model, resulting in drug-addicted sex workers being able to reduce their risk-taking, although not completely as many still require money to 'top up' their prescription. Merseyside is the only area in the UK to prescribe a full range of drugs including heroin, cocaine and amphetamines in a variety of forms (injectable, smokable and oral) on long-term maintenance or reduction. This programme has resulted in over forty women stopping working altogether and has dramatically reduced risk-taking amongst those still working (Lyn Matthews, personal communication). We must offer drug-addicted sex workers adequate and acceptable options. HIV is a much greater threat to our society than drug use. We must therefore ensure that we do everything within our power to enable drug-addicted sex workers to minimise their levels of risk-taking.

The sex industry provides us with an ideal HIV/AIDS education and prevention opportunity. Sex workers are in a position to become health educators with regard to HIV prevention for a vast number of the general public – their clients. However, sex workers must be empowered in order for this to happen. Legal, political and social barriers to this occurring must be removed.

REFERENCES

Alexander, P. (1988) 'Prostitutes are being scapegoated for heterosexual AIDS', in F. Delacoste and P. Alexander (eds) *Sex Work*, London: Virago.

Altman, D. (1988) Report and conference papers, sex industry and AIDS debate. First National Sex Industry Conference, Melbourne, Australia.

Benjamin, H. and Masters, R. (1964) *Prostitution and Morality*, New York: Julian.

Bess, B. and Janus, S. (1976) 'Prostitution', in B.J. Sadock, H.J. Kaplan and A.M. Freedman (eds) *The Sexual Experience*, Baltimore: Williams and Wilkens.

Brown, M. (1979) 'Teenage prostitution', *Adolescence* 14: 665-80.

Bryan, J. (1965) 'Apprenticeships in prostitution', *Social Problems* 12: 287–97.

Bullough, V. (1965) 'Problems and methods for research in prostitution and the behavioural sciences', *Journal of History of Behavioural Sciences* 1: 244–51.

Bullough, V. and Bullough, B. (1978) *Prostitution: An Illustrated Social History*, New York: Crown.

Darrow, W. (1984) 'Prostitution and sexually transmitted diseases', in K.K. Holmes, P.A. Mardh, P.F. Sparling and P.J. Weisner (eds) *Sexually Transmitted Diseases*, McGraw-Hill.

Darrow, W. (1989) 'Prostitutes and their clients'. Unpublished paper from International Workshop: Promoting Safer Sex, Netherlands.

Darrow, W. (1990) 'Assessing targeted AIDS prevention in male and female prostitutes and their clients'. Paper Presented at International Conference: Assessing AIDS Prevention, Montreaux, Switzerland.

Davis, N. (1971) 'The prostitute: developing a deviant identity', in J. Henslin, (ed.) *Studies in the Sociology of Sex*, New York: Appleton-Century-Crofts.

Exner, J., Wylie, J., Leura, A. and Parrill, T. (1977) 'Some psychological characteristics of prostitutes', *Journal of Personality Assessment* 41: 474–85.

Gray, D. (1973) 'Turning out: a study of teenage prostitution', *Urban Life and Culture* 1: 401–25.

Greenwald, H. (1958) *The Call Girl: A Social and Psychoanalytic Study*, New York: Balantine.

Hirschi, T. (1972) 'The professional prostitute', in R. Bell and M. Gordon (eds) *The Social Dimension of Human Sexuality*, Boston: Little Brown.

James, J. (1976) 'Motivations for entrance to prostitution', in L. Crites (ed.) *The Female Offender*, Lexington, MA: Lexington.

Maerov, A. (1965) 'Prostitution: a survey and review of 20 cases', *Psychiatric Quarterly* 39: 675–701.

Morgan Thomas, R., Plant, M.A., Plant, M.L. and Sayles, J. (1990a) 'AIDS-related risks and the sex industry: a Scottish study', Sixth International Conference on AIDS, San Francisco.

Morgan Thomas, R., Plant, M.A., Plant, M.L. and Sayles, D.I. (1990b) 'Risks of AIDS among workers in the "sex industry": some initial results from a Scottish study', *British Medical Journal* 229: 148–9.

Parisot, J. (1987) *Johnny Come Lately: A Short History of the Condom*, London: Journeyman.

Pheterson, G. (1985) *The Whore Stigma: Female Dishonour and Male Unworthiness*, Ministry of Social Affairs and Employment, Netherlands.

Pheterson, G. (1990) 'The category "prostitute" in scientific inquiry', *Journal of Sex Research* 27(3): 397–407.

Polonsky, M. (1974) *The Not-so-happy Hooker: A Psychological Comparison between the Professional Prostitute and Other Women*. Unpublished doctoral dissertation, University of Tennessee, Knoxville.

Potterat, J., Phillips, L., Rotherberg, R. and Darrow, W. (1985) 'On becoming a prostitute: an exploratory case-comparison study', *Journal of Sex Research* 21(3): 329–35.

Visser, J. (1989) 'Policy questions related to HIV and prostitution'. Unpublished paper, World Health Organisation meeting on HIV and prostitution: Interventions.

7 Developing a service for prostitutes in Glasgow

Netta Maciver

Strathclyde Social Work Department currently manages a service for prostitutes which it runs jointly with the Greater Glasgow Health Board. By 1991 over 500 women were using the service. In this chapter I shall look at why such a service was set up in the West of Scotland and how it has developed.

BACKGROUND

Throughout 1986 knowledge was growing about AIDS and HIV and there was increasing concern about the risks, particularly for drug injectors. Information gained from the work of Roy Robertson, a General Practitioner whose practice included a peripheral housing estate in Edinburgh, suggested that up to 50 per cent of drug injectors might be seropositive for HIV (Robertson *et al.* 1986). An uncompleted piece of research postulated that there might be as many as 2,000 drug injectors in Edinburgh (Haw and Liddell 1987). Earlier research (Haw 1985) had suggested that there might be 5,000 drug injectors in Glasgow. According to drug projects and area teams, and from the number of referrals to residential rehabilitation communities, it was clear that drug use had continued to rise since the publication of this research.

Strathclyde Social Work Department, which provides services to a population of almost three million, felt that there was considerable cause for concern. The multidisciplinary group involved in compiling the Department's strategic response to AIDS and HIV suggested that there were between 10,000 and 12,000 drug injectors (Strathclyde Regional Council 1988). It was also known that many female drug injectors raised money for drugs by means of prostitution. They were therefore at risk in two ways – from injecting and from heterosexual spread.

There were a number of factors which contributed to the development of a service for prostitutes. In the absence of a strategic response from the

Scottish Office, Strathclyde Social Work Department initiated a local co-ordinated response which led to the publication of its AIDS and HIV strategy (Strathclyde Regional Council 1988) in December 1988. This contained over a hundred recommendations including one relating to the development of work with male and female prostitutes. This strategy had the approval of four Health Authorities and the full Regional Council.

A further factor was that the Chief Executive of the Regional Council had vested 'lead officer' status in the Director of Social Work. In 1987 he instituted a group of key officers from different Departments of the Council including an Assistant Chief Constable, an Assistant Director of Education and myself. At that time I was Principal Officer (Addiction Services) in Strathclyde Social Work Department. The group was also attended by, amongst others, a Community Medicine Specialist from Greater Glasgow Health Board.

The importance of this group to the development of the service for prostitutes should not be underestimated. It gave me easy and informal access to all Departments of the Council whose help might be required. In particular it contributed to a good working relationship with senior police officers – something not always enjoyed by other such projects. Of additional assistance was the fact that possession of condoms was no longer necessarily to be used as proof of soliciting in Scotland. This meant that a service could be developed without one Regional Department (Social Work) being in conflict with another (the Police).

DEVELOPING THE SERVICE

The initial task of developing the service was given to two Principal Officers: I was responsible for addiction services and a male colleague covered services for offenders. A decision was taken to concentrate initially on women, and in particular on those women who worked on the streets. The first aims were to gather information about services in existence and in use, and to learn more about the number of women who worked. A decision was taken to develop the service from Headquarters rather than pass it out to a District for development. Little was known of what might be required and so it was impossible to draw up a brief at that stage.

The Police Commander for the city centre was indeed a bonus! He was not only prepared to help but was interested in the development. With assistance from him and official records it was estimated that 250 women were working in the city centre. In addition it emerged that there were approximately ten massage parlours in the city. Figures for women working there came later from the women themselves, based on the number of shifts and the number of women working on each shift – a further 250. Contact with health services suggested that some working prostitutes used the services of Genito-Urinary Medicine and of Family Planning but the numbers were negligible.

The next step was to gather information from working prostitutes. To achieve this it was decided to set up a meeting for prostitutes to meet with staff of the Social Work Department to discuss concerns that the women might be at risk of HIV infection. The police offered to help by handing out information about the meeting to women at the point of arrest. Court-based social workers (in Scotland the probation service is part of mainstream social work provision) also passed information to women who appeared before the court on charges of soliciting. Lastly, the social work section in the women's prison gave information to women at the point of discharge from prison. (In Scotland women cannot be imprisoned for soliciting but they *can* be imprisoned for non-payment of fines.)

Although such help was appreciated, it was being delivered at very negative points so we did not anticipate a massive or positive response. Spurred on by the fact that the Director of Social Work intended to attend the first meeting, my colleague and I set out to invite women personally. Street prostitution occurs in one main part of the city centre which is occupied almost entirely by the business community during the day. The police supplied information about the streets in use.

Before setting off we discussed many of our doubts. Could this service contribute to further scapegoating of an already much scapegoated group? Would the service offer something positive or simply contribute to further control? Would the women be exposed to publicity and risk to their family and community lives? It was possible that it could do all of these things. Did we have the right to intrude? Finally, accepting that a service could only proceed as a partnership with the women concerned, we set off. The first two women I approached were extremely helpful, interested and prepared to pass information to others. My male colleague had less success – the women approached took to their heels. Later they explained that he did not appear to be a 'punter' (client) so he had to be a 'vice' (policeman)!

At the first meeting we set ourselves to listen. The women who attended were able to give us information about prostitution and to articulate some of the services which they believed prostitutes needed. They clarified that there were no pimps active in the area, the women having acted together some time before to get rid of them.

With them we arrived at a decision to continue to meet on a regular basis, on a night and at a time which suited them, and in the location which best suited them. It is important to emphasise how few services consider the user of the service as having the right to stipulate these basics.

Meetings were held fortnightly for two hours. Condoms were supplied by the health service (Greater Glasgow Health Board) and distributed by those who attended to others. Information leaflets were gathered from all corners of the globe and discussed for potential value to Glasgow women. Videos about HIV and AIDS were shown. Safer sex and its implementation in the women's working environment formed the basis of many discussions. Many women had horror stories to tell about their use of condoms and still more had misconceptions about how to use them. Discussions frequently concerned partners, child care and the difficulties of running a home and managing a budget. By this time the male officer had changed jobs and two female members of the research staff had joined me. One commented that it reminded her of another women's group that she attended.

Two distinct groups of women emerged. One was an older group of non-drug injectors who had worked as prostitutes for some time. They had rules concerning work and could be harsh in enforcing these but they could be equally supportive to new women in helping them to work more safely. The other group was much younger and had begun to work as prostitutes as a consequence of their drug use. Some were very chaotic in their drug use.

Work was going on simultaneously to obtain finance to set up and run a service. Discussions were held with politicians and many of the other Council departments and there was ongoing consultation with the health authority. Another important colleague came from the Estates Department. As women began to firm up on what they wanted it became clear that premises would be required and it was important that these premises should be easily accessible within the working area. The Estates Department was able to locate premises which had formerly been used as a massage parlour and which had a limited life, making letting difficult and our bid for them more interesting. The owner knew what we planned to operate from the premises and did not question it but forbade the use of the premises as a needle exchange. Some activities are more acceptable than others! A voluntary organisation was already assisting by allowing women to collect condoms from their premises on evenings when there were no meetings. Colleagues from the Health Service had begun to use these premises to offer a direct health service pending the developing of the mainstream service. This was helpful to women in allowing them to decide which services should be on offer in the new premises.

WHAT KIND OF SERVICE?

After one year the outline of what was required was beginning to take shape. Women wanted somewhere they could go to get warm, to have a coffee and a chat. They wanted easy access to free condoms and the services of Genito-Urinary Medicine. They wanted good health care without having to explain what they did. Drug injectors wanted access to rehabilitation when they wanted it. Women needed a place to go for help when attacked during their work, for help with court, fines, welfare rights, housing and violent partners. They needed health care when pregnant and some needed help with child care problems. Nobody wanted a service designed to save them from prostitution!

The service was designed to operate on five evenings per week from 7.30 pm to midnight and was initially staffed by one and a half social work staff. Each evening a doctor or nurse was available for health care with additional staff coming from a variety of settings – drug projects, prison, welfare rights, voluntary bodies. Within months it was clear that the social work staffing had been underestimated and staffing levels were increased. Food was important, particularly for the more chaotic drug injectors, many of whom did not spend money on food. Tea, coffee and cold drinks were provided as were sandwiches, soup, fruit and biscuits. Women were not asked to pay for these.

The service was managed by me together with an advisory group which included a Chief Superintendent of Police, the Health Board's AIDS Co-ordinator, a senior Nursing Officer and two women speaking on behalf of users of the service, one representing non-drug injectors and the other representing the drug injectors. The premises were furnished, staff in post and, following two years of planning, the doors opened in April 1989 to a service jointly supported by the Regional Council and the Health Board. The ultimate test was to come. Would women use the service or would they avoid it, as many agencies had suggested, because it was run by a statutory authority?

In April 1989 51 women used the service 291 times; 36 of them were drug injectors (62 per cent). One year later, during April 1990, 181 women used the service on 899 occasions; 111 were drug injectors (61 per cent). In the first eighteen months 386 women were recorded as having used the service at least once, of whom 226 (59 per cent) were drug injectors, 61 (16 per cent) were non-drug injectors and 99 (26 per cent) were of unknown status. Over 30 attended each evening and newcomers to the service averaged 20 per month.

By the end of 1990 nearly 500 women had used the service and the strains on staff and premises were heavy. The original balance in the group who helped develop the service no longer existed. Drug injectors formed the majority of centre users and non-drug injectors became increasingly unwilling to use the service other than for direct access to condoms, health care and immediate problems. The social element and caring which had earlier been demonstrated had diminished. After discussion with the women it was agreed that when the premises were extended to cope with the increase in numbers, each group would be given time and space from each other. It is to be hoped that this will restore greater tolerance.

SOME DIFFICULT ISSUES

It may be useful to look in some detail at a number of difficult issues which we tried to address.

Rules

Much time was spent in discussion of what rules should apply to users of the service. Anyone who has worked with drug users will know that the more rules that apply the more enterprising will be the attempts to thwart them. That is not to say that drug users are devious characters intent on spoiling the worker's noble intentions! It is rather an acceptance that, for many drug users, procuring and using drugs is the most important activity and relationship that they have. For a worker to feel upset or attacked is pointless. Accordingly it was felt that the fewer rules that applied the better.

Many drug projects have a rule that drug users may only use their service when free from drugs. Such projects usually have primary aims of drug cessation or safer drug use, whereas the primary aim of this service was to allow women to work more safely, thereby protecting themselves, their families and their clients. It did not make sense to exclude those who were intoxicated either from legal or illicit drugs. The outcome of not having such a rule is that there may be women present who are unable to sit, talk or relate in any way. The minimum that is supplied is a safe place for them to be while in that state. Their presence often makes discussion impossible while they are being propped up or helped to avoid burning themselves with hot tea or cigarettes. Other drug users can find this as distressing as the non-drug users. During a consultation exercise with a wide group of users we were asked to request that those 'gouching' on drugs be asked to leave the centre. However, none of the service users were keen to be involved in enforcing this rule.

Whilst accepting that most women will have used drugs prior to coming in or on leaving, there is a rule that no drugs should be used on the premises, and to help enforce this handbags may not be taken into the toilets. This rule is intended to protect the service and is explained to users in this way. Consumption of alcohol on the premises is also forbidden. Although tobacco pollutes the atmosphere so far nobody has suggested that it be banned too! Verbal or physical violence between women or directed towards staff is also forbidden. Respect for each other is encouraged but this is often difficult for a group whose respect for themselves is so low. Use of the telephone for private calls is not allowed but it is available for contact with workers or in relation to particular problems. The trading of goods is also prohibited. Many of these rules must be seen as artificial since women can go outside the door and arrange deals of drugs or stolen goods. The rules are there to safeguard the service.

Once rules have been created, consideration has to be given to what happens when people breach them. Pressure came from users of the service to ban particularly difficult women. Such a ban may be easier to enforce on less likeable characters but is pointless for all concerned. The service is there to safeguard health and therefore should not be denied in order to punish someone. If someone repeatedly breaches rules they are denied access to the social facilities of the service and may only come in to see the medical staff and to collect condoms. In reality it has rarely had to be enforced. The lack of rules forces the staff to consider other ways of controlling behaviour which can be extremely taxing.

Staffing and staff support

Shaping a service to suit its users is likely to attract and sustain good use of the service but is less likely to fall within existing staff conditions of service. Accordingly centre staff are employed on contracts specially designed to suit the service. The centre operates until midnight and it is rarely possible for staff to leave immediately. There can be problems for staff who do not drive since public transport is much reduced after midnight. Staff have to walk through a part of the city which is known as a centre of prostitution and they often attract the attention of kerb crawlers. Once home it can be extremely difficult to unwind and partners are rarely keen to chat at that time. Staff relate taking two to three hours to relax before being able to sleep. Follow-up work may need to be undertaken early the next morning. Staff are expected to work three evenings per week which leaves twenty hours per week for follow-up work, administration, team meetings and supervision.

In addition to two full-time members of staff there are two sessional workers. In advertising for staff a deliberate attempt was made to recruit from as wide a spectrum as possible and this has led to a mixture of qualified and unqualified staff. A decision was taken that women who had ceased working as prostitutes would be eligible to apply. Consequently advertisements are also placed in the centre. Questions are often asked about whether former prostitutes are actually employed. We take the view that to comment on this would invade personal privacy. The worker's previous experience and suitability for the work is confidential to their application form and interview and should not be commented on publicly simply to enhance the employing authority's image.

The service has tended to draw staff who believe that prostitutes are entitled to a service. They believe in enhancing the lives of the women and may enter the service believing that the women have chosen to work as prostitutes and are happy about their choice. In the Glasgow centre the number who are happy with their choice is extremely small. The majority are drug injectors who have become prostitutes because prostitution raises money sufficiently quickly for their drugs and is less likely to lead to imprisonment than shoplifting, housebreaking or mugging.

Drug injectors tend to look down on the non-drug-using prostitutes in the belief that they do not have to prostitute but choose to. Non-drug-using prostitutes look down on the drug users as being captive to drugs and dealers. When asking women for their views on things it is all too common to hear the drug users say 'Don't ask me, I'm only a junkie'.

Women are sometimes raped at work and many are subject to abuse from violent partners. Staff who wish to enhance the quality of life and choice for women find it difficult to cope when women continue to live in degrading circumstances. The stress for staff of being exposed to the levels of pain and suffering experienced by women who come into the centre each evening can be extremely taxing. It appears that the fewer illusions staff have about the glamours of prostitution the better.

It is important to stress that this is the situation found in Glasgow. It should not be taken that this is the definitive picture of prostitution in Scotland or in the United Kingdom. There are a small number of women who work to supplement family income and quality of life. They work specific hours and are clear about what they will tolerate from clients and others. They are a tiny minority of the women who work in Glasgow.

The implications for staff support and stress management are clear but are less simple to resolve. How do you help staff to relax at 2 a.m.? How do you help a member of staff to accept the depressing reality of working with someone who at this point does not wish to change their drug use or their violent partner? Equally depressing for staff is the reality that most drug-injecting HIV positive women will continue to work even when ill. Neither illness nor the knowledge of oncoming death stops the determined drug injector from further drug use and, in the absence of substitute drugs on prescription, from further prostitution to finance their street drugs. Staff believe that for some extremely ill women the system needs to provide a range of injectables on prescription.

At the time of writing the centre is at an early stage in resolving any of these staff support issues and various types of staff support have been tried, including stress management techniques, individual supervision and team supervision.

Record-keeping and confidentiality

The sceptics had told us that women would not come to a service run by the Social Work Department because of their fears about the controls the Department could exercise in respect of their children. Staff concerns focused on how much information they would have to pass to social work teams in order to comply with the Department's child care procedures. The women helping to develop the service were worried that the Department would build up documentation about them which might be used in some other context. We agreed that a record-keeping system was essential in only two contexts: first, it needed to record the use of the service and how the demands on it changed and, second, when staff were involved in referring on individuals, they needed to keep documentation concerning the referral. The system devised emerged from a re-statement of the aim of the service, i.e. it exists to provide a direct health and social service to working prostitutes. It does not aim to provide an individual casework service to women but can act as an important referral point to other agencies and sectors of the Department. Women using the service give a first name and are given a number. They are asked whether or not they are drug injectors. Each night an attendance sheet is available and women sign in with their name and number. This has allowed research staff to develop a system which provides monthly feedback to staff and managers of the service.

If a woman requests individual help she provides her name and address for referral purposes and is asked permission for the information to be passed on. It is not intended that centre staff continue on a co-worker basis although there have been times when this has happened with the consent of the women.

Problems occur when other social workers want information from centre staff on whether women still use the service. This information is not divulged. The centre is not in a monitoring role in respect of women's behaviour. In child care cases when social workers have lost contact with women and there are child care interests, information can be passed to women to encourage them to re-establish contact but the decision to do so can only be theirs. If the centre were to become a monitoring point for other workers then women would cease to trust it and use it. Centre staff often feel that they are in an invidious position in respect of fieldwork colleagues who may be looking for proof in child care cases. They also feel that some colleagues have negative views about prostitution. Prostitutes span the range of child care abilities and they may be good, mediocre or poor parents. The quality of these abilities is for fieldworkers with their assessment skills to determine. Centre staff who do not see the women with their children are not in a position to contribute to such an assessment.

Contact with the press

The developing service came under scrutiny from the press at an early stage. Strathclyde Social Work Department prides itself on having an open relationship with the press but the developing service was not owned solely by the Department. The women who attended therefore had to have some say in press involvement. They were given the right to veto any article and staff working with them tried to encourage them to use the press constructively, to say what they wanted to say. They learned to ask for earlier articles and to evaluate the articles that had been written by journalists with whom they had co-operated.

Research

Researchers were also extremely interested in the women. The main purpose of the initiative however was to provide a service. Research was necessary to learn more about the problems women faced, in order to further shape the service, but all involved agreed that research should not supersede service provision. The research staff involved planned and administered questionnaires and women participated well. Women were told in advance when research was scheduled so that they could choose whether or not to participate.

These are some of the issues encountered in setting up the centre for prostitutes in Glasgow. Different areas may meet other or additional problems.

CONCLUSION

There was a great deal of satisfaction in being able to create and shape the service along with those who would go on to use it. It is important that such centres should not develop a set or rigid way of doing things but should always keep themselves open to changing demand. In this way they should avoid becoming a club for those who are current users while newcomers look on, wondering how they join. The provision needs to retain a fresh outlook, tuned to client need, and able and willing to change when required. Change should not be seen as a criticism of what exists but as a demonstration of a flexible approach.

The drop-in centre for prostitutes in Glasgow came into existence because of the high level of commitment to such a service by senior officers within the Social Work Department and benefited enormously from the easy access to senior colleagues in other Departments. It has become a well-used service because its main architects are the women who use it. It will continue in existence and hopefully expand because of this shared commitment and because of the willingness of the local authority politicians to provide it as a mainstream service.

REFERENCES

Haw, S.J. (1985) *Drug Problems in Greater Glasgow*, London: SCODA.

Haw, S.J. and Liddell, D. (1987) *Drug Addiction in Edinburgh District: Report of the SCODA Fieldwork Survey*, London: SCODA.

Robertson, J.R., Bucknall, A.B.V., Welsby, P.D., Roberts, J.J.K., Inglis, J.M., Peutherer, J.F. and Brettle, R.P. (1986) 'Epidemic of AIDS-related virus (HTLV–III/LAV) infection among intravenous drug abusers', *British Medical Journal* 242: 527–9.

Strathclyde Regional Council (1988) *HIV Infection and AIDS: Towards an Inter-agency Strategy.*

Part IV

Education and counselling issues

8 Education and the prevention of HIV infection

Judy Bury

At face value the prevention of HIV infection seems simple. It has even been suggested that not one more person needs to become infected with HIV. The prevention message is certainly very clear:

- avoid intercourse if you can; if you must have intercourse, use a condom.
- don't inject drugs; if you must inject, don't share needles and syringes.

So what is the problem? Why is prevention difficult? Obviously this is an issue for both men and women but in this chapter I shall explore some of the reasons why prevention is more difficult than it seems, concentrating particularly on why *women* find it difficult to protect themselves against HIV infection. I shall then go on to look at some of the implications of this for sex education in schools.

My own experience has been as a doctor and counsellor in a youth advisory centre and subsequently as a general practitioner, during which time I also visited schools to talk about relationships, sex and contraception. I have had less involvement in health education but I shall discuss some of the issues that seem to me to be important in mass media health campaigns. I shall also look at some implications for counselling women at risk.

DIFFICULTIES WITH HIV PREVENTION

One factor that affects people's willingness to protect themselves is the extent to which they perceive themselves to be at risk (Aggleton *et al.* 1988, Stockdale *et al.* 1989). Much irresponsible journalism, fuelled by pronouncements by some public figures, has led many people to believe that the risk of heterosexual transmission of HIV infection is very small. The continuing tendency to talk of 'high risk groups' and to attribute blame, has led many people to think that AIDS is something that happens to other people and not to them (Aggleton *et al.* 1988). Thus heterosexual people may convince themselves that AIDS affects only homosexuals, while those who do not use drugs may see AIDS as affecting only drug users.

Along with this goes a reluctance to identify as belonging to a group that is seen to be at risk (Abrams *et al.* 1990). Thus someone who only occasionally injects may not identify as a drug user, and a woman who identifies as a lesbian yet occasionally has sex with men may not think of herself as being at risk. A woman who has numerous sexual partners may see AIDS as something that happens to people who are 'promiscuous' or to prostitutes, and not to someone like herself.

Even when women acknowledge that they are at risk, there are a number of reasons why they do not find it easy to persuade men to use condoms, or to use a barrier such as a diaphragm or spermicide themselves. Just as some women find it difficult to use contraception to prevent pregnancy, so, for similar reasons, some women find it difficult to use barriers to prevent transmission of HIV infection.

Probably the most important factor affecting women's use of contraception or protection is their attitude to their own sexuality. Many women find it difficult to accept themselves as sexual. They may want to have sex and yet they may have been brought up to believe that women should not want to have sex but should be passive in a sexual relationship – sex is something that happens *to* them and they are not responsible for what happens. One young woman interviewed after attending a clinic for the first time described this dilemma:

> We all have a moralistic background that prevents us from admitting to ourselves that we are likely to have intercourse until it actually happens. So it's impossible to go on the pill beforehand because that would be admitting that you are wanting to have sex. We're prevented by our background from admitting that.
>
> (McGlew *et al.* 1989)

This ambivalence about sexuality may make it difficult to use contraception and especially to be prepared for sex by having contraception available (McGlew *et al.* 1989).

If a woman uses a barrier, this will prevent pregnancy as well as transmission of infection, yet many women may not be clear about wanting to prevent pregnancy. Many young women, especially those who feel that they have no prospects for achieving anything fulfilling in their lives, may see pregnancy as a desirable option or at least may not feel that there is much incentive for them to prevent pregnancy. Having a child may feel like the only creative thing that they can do (Bury 1984).

For women with HIV infection, the incentive to have a baby may be even greater (see Chapters 2 and 4). A woman who is not infected herself but has an infected partner may be caught between wanting to protect herself from infection and wanting to have a child with this man whom she loves. Thus, women may accept that they should not become pregnant because of the risks but may be swayed by other emotions that make pregnancy seem attractive. Such ambivalence about pregnancy makes it very difficult to use barrier contraception reliably even though this would offer protection against infection.

Many young women lack self-esteem. This contributes to their ambivalence about pregnancy but it also makes it difficult for them to assert themselves with their partner and insist that he use a condom for protection. Women tend to lack power in relationships and what happens sexually is often determined by men (Holland *et al.* 1990). Women may fear the repercussions of taking a stand about contraception and protection, let alone suggesting that they should avoid intercourse.

Many people, especially those living in deprived areas, may feel that they have little control over their lives, that there are many outside forces that determine their future. They may find it difficult to take action to determine their own future, taking a fatalistic attitude to their lives and health. This affects the ability of many people to act on messages about health promotion. The ability of some young women to use contraception effectively to prevent pregnancy is one example of this (Bury 1984). Similarly they may not be able to protect themselves from HIV infection by practising safer sex.

Lack of self-esteem and the feeling of lack of control also affect the ability of drug users, both men and women, to accept and act on the prevention message about not sharing needles. Another factor that makes this difficult is the tendency of many drug users to behave as adolescents, whatever their age. Like adolescents, they may be impulsive, they may feel invulnerable and live for the moment, looking for immediate gratification and they may find it difficult to think in terms of consequences. All this may make it difficult for them to stick to one course of action for any length of time and tends to lead to risk-taking behaviour in relation to the prevention of HIV infection as in many other areas of their lives. Most drug users eventually mature out of this behaviour. What has been striking is that, even at a stage when still using drugs and when still behaving chaotically in many aspects of their lives, many injecting drug users, men and women, *have* stopped injecting whilst those who continue to inject have been able to reduce their needle-sharing to a great extent (Stimson *et al.* 1988). Although many have changed their drug-using behaviour there has been no significant change in sexual behaviour. Clearly changes in sexual behaviour are more difficult for everyone to achieve.

Another factor that makes protection against HIV infection difficult is the problem of safer sex in long-term relationships. A couple may successfully negotiate discussion about previous risks and about protection at the beginning of a relationship but once the relationship has been established for a while, and perhaps both partners have been tested and found to be uninfected, there is usually an assumption that protection is no longer necessary as continuing mutual fidelity is assumed. For a woman to insist on the continued use of condoms is to imply that her partner has been or might be unfaithful. She may fear rejection or even violence. In a longstanding relationship that predates knowledge about AIDS it may be even more difficult to raise the subject of AIDS, condoms and non-penetrative sex. 'For many women... the fear of becoming HIV infected is insignificant in comparison to the fear of reprisal involved in even suggesting to their lovers that they use condoms' (ACT UP 1991).

IMPLICATIONS FOR SEX EDUCATION IN SCHOOLS

As we have seen, many of the factors that affect the ability of young people to use contraception to prevent pregnancy also affect their ability to protect themselves against HIV infection. Although there is general agreement, including agreement from most parents, that school is an appropriate place to teach children about sex, sex education in schools has, up to now, had little impact on the teenage pregnancy rate. Teenagers continue to cite friends and magazines, rather than school, as their main sources of sex education. Although the implications of HIV and AIDS for sex education in schools are not new, they have rarely been put into practice – and there is now an added impetus to get it right.

There is general agreement that HIV/AIDS education should 'take place within the context of sex education which should itself be part of personal, social and health education' (Massey 1987). As nearly half of young people are now likely to have sexual intercourse before the age of 16 years (Bowie and Ford 1989), such education needs to begin before this, at age 13–14 years, needs to be repeated at regular intervals to reinforce the message, and needs to be relevant to each age group. Too often sex education begins too late, after young people have already initiated sexual relationships.

It is essential that the objectives of sex education be realistic. There seems little likelihood that education will have much effect on the small proportion of teenagers who have numerous partners (Ford and Morgan 1989) but there is some reason to believe that it might be possible to encourage the majority of teenagers to wait longer before having intercourse, to get to know their partners better and to have fewer partners (Seltzer *et al.* 1989). It might also be possible to encourage sexually active young men to use condoms and young women to insist on their use but it seems less likely that young people can be encouraged to choose not to have penetrative intercourse (Holland *et al.* 1990).

In many schools sex education continues to take the form of one or two factual lectures. It has long been known that the acquisition of knowledge in any area of health education is not sufficient to change behaviour and, similarly, a number of studies have shown a gulf between knowledge and behaviour in relation to HIV and AIDS (e.g. Brown *et al.* 1987, Reader *et al.* 1988). Thus the simple provision of factual information is not enough. Information needs to be presented in a personally relevant way and young people need to have the opportunity to discuss the issues raised in small groups so that they can clarify their own values and attitudes and can begin to understand how the information relates to them as individuals (Ford and Bowie 1988).

Young people need the opportunity to develop skills in making relationships and need encouragement to make choices about their sexual lifestyle while having due regard for the feelings of others. They need to learn that their choices can change over time and that even if they have had intercourse, they can choose not to continue. As mentioned earlier, one cause of the gap between knowledge and behaviour is that women have less control in sexual encounters, so they have limited ability to control risks (Holland *et al.* 1990). Young women need encouragement to be more assertive in relationships so that they can 'express their own sexual desires and have these met in safety' (Holland *et al.* 1990). Young men need encouragement to talk about sex and relationships and to take on more responsibility for contraception and protection.

It is essential that HIV/AIDS education moves away from a focus on 'high risk groups' to a stance that encourages all young people to consider how they might be at risk and how this risk can be avoided (Clift *et al.* 1987). Yet such education also needs to acknowledge the appeal for young people of risk-taking in relation to sex as in other areas of their lives (Smith 1989). Holland and her colleagues (1990) have pointed out that 'young people can be attracted to the risks of sexual activity by the lure of rebellion. If a particular activity is forbidden, especially by authority, it can become more enticing for some young people.'

Sex educators need to create a safe environment for young people to talk about their sexuality, including the opportunity to explore their concerns about their sexual orientation and the implications that this has for protection against HIV infection. It is important not to exclude, let alone alienate, young people who feel attracted to people of the same sex by ignoring their needs and concerns. Gay teenagers also need sex education that is personally relevant to them.

Sex education in general needs to be more explicit (Holland *et al.* 1990) and to include more discussion. This could include more open discussion about the variety and pleasures of non-penetrative forms of sexual activity combined with practical strategies for raising the issue of safer sex with a partner both at the beginning of a relationship and in long-term relationships. Here again discussion in small groups is essential and both single sex and mixed discussion groups can be helpful.

The quality of sex education tends to depend on the willingness and skill of the staff who are involved. It also depends on the quality of personal contact on a day-to-day basis. There needs to be more emphasis on training and support for teachers in this area of the curriculum (Royal College of Obstetricians and Gynaecologists 1991).

Sex education strategies may benefit from the involvement of health professionals (Abrams *et al.* 1990) but it is important that HIV/AIDS education does not become isolated from other aspects of the curriculum. It can be actively built in to many subjects, for example by using literature which has AIDS as a theme in English and by looking at issues that are raised by the pandemic in geography and modern studies. Young people need encouragement to raise issues related to HIV and AIDS in these and many other contexts (Massey 1987). It is also important that parents are given the opportunity to discuss the sex education programme that is planned and to see the materials that will be used (Massey 1987). This helps to defuse anxiety and destroy myths about the dangers of responsible sex education. For example, parents can be reassured that sex education does not encourage young people to experiment with sex. On the contrary, sex education has the potential to encourage young people to act with more responsibility in their relationships (Bury 1984). Consultation with parents can lead to support for innovative approaches relevant to that community.

MASS MEDIA CAMPAIGNS

Given the difficulty that women have in protecting themselves against HIV infection, it is interesting that so much attention is focused on women in mass media campaigns. From many of the posters and advertisements that have been produced, it would seem that women are expected to take responsibility for protecting themselves *and* protecting men. Much health education effort has been directed at women to persuade them that it is *their* responsibility to get men to use condoms.

There is obviously some justification for this from a historical perspective. Women have always had to protect themselves against pregnancy and disease. Sometimes men shared in this responsibility but since the advent of the pill there have been nearly thirty years during which the use of the condom has declined and there is now a whole generation of men who have handed over to women the responsibility for preventing pregnancy. During this time sexually transmitted diseases were gradually forgotten as they were seen as treatable.

With the advent of AIDS, rather than trying to persuade men to use condoms once again, the attention has focused mostly on women. Support for this approach came from research in the latter half of the 1980s (Health Education Authority 1988) which showed that women took the risk of AIDS more seriously than men and were easier to convince of the need for safer sex.

This research was the justification for the Health Education Authority campaign during the late 1980s which targeted women with the intention of: 'alerting women to the risk of HIV infection and providing them with the motivation, information and confidence to avoid it' (Health Education Authority 1989). The aim of the campaign was: 'to encourage women to discuss condom use with their partners and to help them [that is, the women] feel they have the confidence to take appropriate action' (Health Education Authority 1989).

The campaign produced newspaper and magazine advertisements that were clearly directed at women with slogans such as 'She's too embarrassed to ask him to use a condom' and 'Is this... um, how you'd... well, feel about... er, asking your boyfriend to... um... well... er... use a condom?'

It may be *understandable* that so much of the campaign has been directed at women, reinforcing their role in taking responsibility and letting men off the hook, but I believe that it is not only unreasonable, in that it continues to place too much of the burden on women, but it is also counterproductive. It ignores the fact that ultimately it is the man that must use the condom and it is the man that must be persuaded that it is the right thing to do to protect himself as well as the woman. To give women the sole responsibility ignores the problems that women have in even raising the subject of condoms, let alone demanding that their partners use one. It ignores the lack of power that most women feel in determining the type of sexual activity engaged in (Holland *et al.* 1990). It also ignores the attitude that a woman who carries condoms is looking for casual sex and is to be derided as a 'slag' (Lees 1986).

The prevention of HIV infection relies on the condom or the avoidance of penetrative sex, both of which rely on the co-operation of men. Just as the prevention of pregnancy became more efficient when women gained access to the pill, a method that women controlled, it is also likely that the prevention of HIV infection would become more efficient if there were effective methods available to women (Anonymous 1990, Stein 1990). Yet the research needed to investigate the safety of existing spermicides and to develop new spermicides or other new female methods has not been properly funded.

It is essential that we work towards changing the attitudes that make it difficult for women to carry condoms and the power relationships that make it difficult for women to insist on their use but we also need to acknowledge that this is going to take a long time. In the meantime, we need to *inform* women of the risk of HIV infection and *support* them in their continuing need to act responsibly, but we also need to start to *persuade* men to take some share in the responsibility too. Otherwise we are in danger of producing yet another generation of men who leave the responsibility to women. Surely the prevention of HIV infection, like the prevention of pregnancy, should become a shared responsibility?

This kind of approach is not impossible. Some posters have been produced in Britain and elsewhere that simply set out to inform women of the risk of HIV infection, with slogans such as 'Women can get AIDS too'. There have also been some efforts to produce posters directed at both men and women, for example a poster promoting condom use with the slogan 'Women's self-defence and men's responsibility'. This approach also underlies the 'Take Care Campaign' in Lothian which promotes the message 'take care of the one you love' and focuses equally on men and women.

For health education campaigns to be effective, those targeted need to 'see the messages as relevant to themselves as individuals' (Stockdale *et al.* 1989). As long as heterosexuals continue to see AIDS as something that happens to other people, they are unlikely to change their behaviour. Mass media campaigns may need to target those who are particularly vulnerable such as those who are not in a stable relationship (Stockdale *et al.* 1989).

TARGETING WOMEN AT RISK

Some women are particularly at risk of HIV infection, such as prostitutes, women who inject drugs and women with partners who may be infected. One of the major difficulties is how to target such women. A great deal has been done to inform and support prostitutes so that they can protect themselves (see Chapters 6 and 7). But women at particular risk of HIV infection are all different – apart from being at risk and being women, they may not have much else in common. They are difficult to target and, if they are targeted in mass media campaigns, this may increase the stigma. What is particularly worrying is that many women do not even realise that they are at risk.

It is important to emphasise that mass media campaigns are not the most effective means of reaching specific groups in the population. Alternative approaches need to be employed such as peer education (see Chapter 6) and outreach. Those working with women need to take the opportunity to tell them about the risks of needle-sharing and also have a responsibility to tell them the facts about heterosexual transmission (see Chapter 4 and Table 8.1).

Giving people the facts is not enough; education needs to be a two-way

Table 8.1 The facts about heterosexual transmission

1	Contrary to what is sometimes claimed, you can catch HIV through vaginal intercourse.
2	It may be slightly easier for a man to infect a woman than for a woman to infect a man, but both can happen.
3	You can catch HIV from one act of intercourse – and there are now several documented cases of this happening.
4	You can't tell by looking at someone whether they are infected – and they may not know themselves if they are infected.
5	Although there may be times when people with HIV infection are more infectious than at other times, there is no time when it is safe to have unprotected intercourse with someone who is infected.
6	You may have unprotected intercourse repeatedly with someone who is HIV positive without getting infected but that doesn't mean you're safe – or immune – you may get infected the very next time. This is particularly dangerous as your infected partner begins to get ill as their infectiousness may increase at this time.
7	If your sexual partner is infected it is best to avoid penetration if you can. If you must have intercourse, use a condom – and if that's not possible, use a spermicide.

process. It is important to check that the factual information is understood. Encouraging people to avoid penetrative sex is particularly difficult. It is not easy to get over to a couple that sex without penetration can be fun. It is even more difficult to help a woman to negotiate non-penetrative sex with her partner when you are only seeing her. It is essential to talk to the men too.

Women with HIV-infected partners are faced with the prospect of having to practice safer sex indefinitely and this can be very daunting. If they decide to have a child they then have the added problem of trying to get pregnant while limiting the risk of becoming infected (see Chapter 4).

SOME IMPLICATIONS FOR COUNSELLING

Given the factors that make it difficult for women to protect themselves against HIV infection and to respond to educational messages, there is a need for sensitive counselling to help people to address these issues and to take on board what they have learned. It is not enough just to tell people 'use a condom' or 'don't share needles'. Counsellors need to help women to recognise their ambivalence about sexuality and pregnancy and to acknowledge some of the other difficulties that they may have in putting prevention into practice.

Many counsellors have experienced the frustration of knowing a woman who continues to have unprotected intercourse with her partner whom she knows to be infected. Exhortation to use condoms is not enough. I have found that it is important to ask *why* a woman finds it difficult to get her partner to use condoms and to listen to the answer. A woman consulted me whose partner was HIV positive but they were continuing to have unprotected intercourse. I asked her why. She told me that when he had been told that he was HIV positive he had been very distressed and had worried that no-one would love him any more and that no-one would come near him. He felt unclean. She felt unable to ask him to use condoms – to put a barrier between him and her – as she felt that he would interpret this as rejection, as a sign that she no longer loved him. We discussed other ways for her to show him that she loved him and discussed and tried out ways that she could ask him to use condoms. This was a more productive approach than just further exhortation. She has since talked to her partner and they are now using condoms.

Education about the prevention of HIV infection has to be based on an understanding of the factors that make such prevention difficult. Grasping the nettle of planning effective education about HIV prevention could lead to exciting developments in sex education, health education and in counselling. It could also save lives.

REFERENCES

Abrams, D., Abraham, C., Spears, R. and Marks, D. (1990) 'AIDS invulnerability: relationships, sexual behaviour and attitudes among 16–19-year-olds', in P. Aggleton, P. Davies, and G. Hart (eds) *AIDS: Individual, Cultural and Policy Dimensions*, London: Falmer Press.

ACT UP (1991) *Treatment and Research Agenda for Women with HIV Infection*, US: AIDS Coalition to Unleash Power.

Aggleton, P., Homans, H. and Warwick, I. (1988) 'Young people, sexuality education and AIDS', *Youth and Policy* 23: 5–13.

Anonymous (1990) 'Barriers and boundaries', *Lancet* 335: 1497–8.

Bowie, C. and Ford, N. (1989) 'Sexual behaviour of young people and the risk of HIV infection', *Journal of Epidemiology and Community Health* 43: 61–5.

Brown, J.S., Irwin, W.G., Steele, K. and Harland, R.W. (1987) 'Students' awareness of and attitudes to AIDS', *Journal of the Royal College of General Practitioners* 37: 457–8.

Bury, J.K. (1984) *Teenage Pregnancy in Britain*, London: Birth Control Trust.

Clift, S., Stears, D. and Legg, S. (1987) 'AIDS education strategies for young people', *Education and Health* 5:108–11.

Ford, N. and Bowie, C. (1988) 'Sexually related behaviour and AIDS education', *Education and Health* 6(4): 86–91.

Ford, N. and Morgan, K. (1989) 'Heterosexual lifestyles of young people in an English city', *Journal of Population and Social Studies* 1(2): 167–82.

Health Education Authority (1988) 'Qualitative research into a proposed AIDS campaign for the women's press', conducted by Reflexions Market Research Ltd. Unpublished report.

Health Education Authority (1989) Circular letter launching women's campaign.

Holland, J., Ramazanoglu, C. and Scott, S. (1990) *Sex, Risk and Danger: Tensions between Government AIDS Education Policy and Young Women's Sexuality*, London: Tufnell Press.

Lees, S. (1986) *Losing Out: Sexuality and Adolescent Girls*, London: Hutchinson.

McGlew, T., Bury, J.K. and Jamieson, L. (1989) *Rationality, Risk Taking and Advice Seeking Amongst New Clients at a Contraceptive Advisory Service*, Edinburgh: Brook Advisory Centre (unpublished manuscript).

Massey, D.E. (1987) 'Teaching about AIDS in schools', *Health Education Journal* 46(2): 66–8.

Reader, E.G., Carter, R.P. and Crawford, A. (1988) 'AIDS – knowledge, attitudes and behaviour: a study with university students', *Health Education Journal* 47(4): 125–7.

Royal College of Obstetricians and Gynaecologists (1991) *Report of the RCOG Working Party on Unplanned Pregnancy*, London: RCOG.

Seltzer, V. L., Rabin, J. and Benjamin, F. (1989) 'Teenagers' awareness of the acquired immunodeficiency syndrome and the impact on their sexual behaviour', *Obstetrics and Gynaecology* 74(1): 55–9.

Smith, M. (1989) 'How children and young people cope with what they know about AIDS', in M. Smith and G. Harding *Health Education and Young People: AIDS and Other Health Related Knowledge*, Occasional Paper No. 9, London: Thomas Coram Research Unit.

Stein, Z.A. (1990) 'HIV prevention: the need for methods women can use', *American Journal of Public Health* 80: 460–2.

Stimson, G.V., Alldritt, L.J., Dolan, K., Donoghue, M.C. and Lart, R.A. (1988) *Injecting Equipment Exchange Schemes*, Final Report for the Department of Health and Social Security and Scottish Home and Health Department, London: Goldsmiths College.

Stockdale, J.E., Dockrell, J.E. and Wells, A.J. (1989) 'The self in relation to mass media representations of HIV and AIDS – match or mismatch?' *Health Education Journal* 48(3): 121–30.

9 Offering safer sex counselling to women from drug-using communities

Jane Wilson

The advent of HIV and AIDS has affected everyone. In drug-using communities the impact on women is particularly acute. They are especially vulnerable, as both users and sexual partners of users, and they also carry the burden of possibly passing on the virus to their children.

Initially it was hoped that education and information about the virus would activate changes in behaviour. It has become increasingly evident that, while the basic facts about HIV transmission are known, the expected corresponding behaviour changes, especially the adoption of safer sex practices by women, have not occurred.

Issues for women around sexuality, pregnancy, self-esteem, and control in their lives have undermined the efficacy and success of HIV/AIDS education in this arena (see Chapter 8). Many women have contradictory feelings about their sexuality, perhaps desiring sex but feeling that they should be passive in sexual relationships. Being prepared for sex by using contraception means accepting that they are sexual and interested in sex. Women often express ambivalence about pregnancy, seeing it as the only creative thing they can do, and therefore are swayed by other emotions that make pregnancy seem attractive despite the risks or sacrifices that may be involved. Along with this, many young women have low self-esteem and feelings of lack of control over their lives, which foster neither assertiveness in sexual relationships nor an ability to negotiate safer sex.

In counselling women about safer sex it would seem that counsellors have a dual role. They must not only provide education and information about HIV and AIDS but, more importantly, they need to address the complex task of engaging women in counselling in order to examine and address the psychosocial factors which often precipitate, sustain and reinforce their current unsafe, high risk sexual practices.

As yet, we can prevent very little if they're not talking to us! Although most women approach our drug counselling service for help with their drug problems, they tend to focus initially on problems of a practical nature such as housing, benefits or court appearances. Requesting counselling for emotional concerns is rarely given as the presenting issue.

In this chapter I shall concentrate on two issues: barriers *to* counselling and barriers *within* counselling which may prevent women from receiving the services they require to take care of themselves in the face of this epidemic. Clearly some of these barriers apply to men as well but it is the specific way in which they apply to women that is of interest to us here.

BARRIERS TO COUNSELLING

Distrust and hostility towards professions and authority

There may be a class bias in the counselling offered. Most trained counsellors are 'middle class' whereas women from drug-using communities are predominantly 'working class'. Counsellors may well experience themselves as having both personal and professional power which is socially legitimated. The women being counselled, however, quite often experience themselves as extremely powerless on both a personal and social level.

It is important that counsellors are sensitive to both cultural and class issues and continually reassess their assumptions and practice to minimise biases which could hamper the counselling work.

Disregard for the counselling process

The value and status of counselling in these communities may easily be superseded by other needs. Talking to a professional counsellor about problems is often seen as a sign of major failure and an inability to cope. My experience in the community has been that this also breaks the unwritten law of taking personal business outside the family. Women may fear that they will be seen as 'crazy' or 'hysterical' if they are referred to or seek some form of counselling. More significantly, talking about problems is seen as an abstract, symbolic process whereas survival in these communities is concrete. Practical assistance in the form of benefits, food vouchers and decent housing are valued far more than seeing a counsellor. For women, counselling can be particularly problematic in that it raises the question of needs. Women have traditionally focused away from exploring or expressing their needs. They have also been socially encouraged to transform their own real needs and see them as identical to or less important than those of others, usually men and children.

I have found it useful in my work to take time in the early sessions to explain in a clear way what the counselling process is about and to set a framework within which the counselling will take place.

Shame, fear and guilt

It is still seen as more socially reprehensible for women than for men to be dependent on illicit drugs, as this jeopardises their role as society's carers (Dorn *et al*. 1991). Coming forward and identifying themselves as drug users may intensify their sense of failure. If there are children involved, a woman may not only feel intense guilt over not achieving the socially acceptable standard of mothering but she may also be very afraid that if she discusses her drug use or that of her partner, her children may be placed on a supervision order or taken away from her.

Playing on a woman's guilt to stimulate change by saying for example 'Think of your kids' or 'Do it for your children's sake' may only increase her sense of shame and guilt. Approaching the problem from the understanding that she cares for and loves her children very much and must be struggling and suffering quite a bit at the times when she is unable to cope with them, may offer her a way to keep some dignity and self-esteem which is fundamental for positive change.

Resistance to involvement

In my experience drug users generally tend to engage in distance-creating manoeuvres to protect themselves from involvement and to avoid getting close to and trusting another person. Women drug users, in particular, may have internalised the social condemnation of their behaviour and may therefore be even more resistant to coming forward. Given that many drug agencies still design and develop services in response to the stereotypic young male user, women often feel out of place if they attempt to use these services. Rather than risk exposure they will remain more acutely isolated.

Approach/avoidance conflict

Drug users will often adopt testing and challenging behaviour to gauge the counsellor's capacity to cope with their feelings of emotional dependency. To engage in the counselling process may mean that, if they open up and begin to explore the extent of their emotional dependency, they may feel too overwhelmed and exposed to survive and may need to close down and withdraw contact. Although society often encourages emotional dependency in women (Miller 1976), many women feel the need to suppress the extent of their abandonment and dependency feelings and remain trapped in 'get closer/pull away' manoeuvres.

Counsellors can sometimes be seduced into feeling that dependency on them by a client will strengthen their position to influence changes they see as beneficial. This can be a shortcut that often backfires, resulting in clients feeling resentful and controlled. While acknowledging that the client has many unmet needs is important, it is equally important that counsellors credit and reflect back to the women each and every way they have made even the smallest positive decision about their lives.

Any combination of these barriers can present as the first wall of resistance and will need to be both recognised and acknowledged if counsellors hope to do effective work. If these barriers can be overcome there are often further problems which arise once counselling begins.

BARRIERS WITHIN COUNSELLING

Conflicts can arise in the counselling process which, if not understood and addressed, can sabotage any fruitful work attempted in the area of preventative counselling. Feelings and reactions to these feelings can be expected from both the counsellor as well as the client. However, they can be easily overlooked or ignored by the counsellor and thus interfere considerably in the outcome.

It is usual for both counsellor and client to have some anxiety about the counselling session at the start. For the counsellor, this often takes the form of generalised concern about the AIDS epidemic, pressure to educate and counsel on prevention and a desire to achieve behavioural change where required. For the client, there may be apprehension about the session itself, concern about what information she may be given and how it affects her personally, and anxiety about what may be expected or requested of her.

Initially, a counsellor's anxiety can be contained or reduced by the structured use of the educative component of the counselling, e.g. presenting the basic facts about HIV/AIDS, assessing the level of risk and offering advice about harm reduction strategies. The client, however, may become increasingly anxious during the course of the session because the information offered does not appear helpful. On one level most women can understand the facts about how to practise safer sex but at a deeper level many women I have worked with have felt that they could not follow through and adopt these practices for reasons they did not understand. They simply keep repeating, often to themselves, 'I just can't do that'. They can begin to feel bad about themselves. If the feelings evoked by this dilemma remain unexplored, the counsellor could be feeding the client's sense of inadequacy, rather than enhancing her sense of competence.

At such a point one can expect the client's resistance to surface either in the form of outright rejection of the counsellor or passive compliance. Defences/barriers will be activated to maintain an already fragile sense of self, and negative feelings that may have been elicited will need to be projected. These defences may be expressed in the following ways:

Denial:	'The government is just trying to scare users.'
Rationalisation:	'My friend's been sleeping with someone who's positive for two years and she's OK, so I'll be fine too.'
Avoidance:	'I'm sorry I missed the last two sessions but...'
	'I can't really stay but I just need to use the phone 'cos my giro didn't come and someone bust my window and my man is gonna batter me and...'
	'I've just got my script and I've taken all my tablets so if I doze off...'

When the client's defences are in operation, this can also have an effect on the counsellor. She can begin to feel ineffectual and inadequate for the task and goal she may have set for herself. She too will need to be aware of negative or uncomfortable feelings which she might experience as a result of her sense of failure or frustration. If not thoroughly worked through in supervision or consultation, the counsellor's own defence system may be activated and begin to interfere in the work. Often this can happen without the counsellor being aware of it and may take the form of:

Rationalisation:	'This is an unmotivated and very difficult client.'
Displacement:	'If only the other person/GP/Social worker/drug service would do their job properly with this woman.'
Avoidance:	'This client has problems that really should be dealt with by that specialist agency.'

Feelings of failure can therefore be experienced by both counsellor and client. For the client, however, negative attitudes about counselling can be reinforced if she becomes stuck on this merry-go-round, and this can leave her feeling more helpless and alone than before she began counselling.

If we approach safer sex counselling fully understanding that the optimal suggestions for safer sex can be experienced by the client as unachievable, and we are able to acknowledge this with the client, we can create an opportunity for working on a 'harm reduction model' on this issue. Asking the client to assess how much she feels at risk, exploring all the options available for increasing her safety, allowing the client to choose what she feels able to manage, even if it is a less safe option (e.g. using a contraceptive sponge permeated with nonoxynol–9), and affirming and supporting her in achieving this, can avoid the dilemma I have described and set the basis for a workable relationship between counsellor and client.

However, along with the emotional confusion which can arise in counselling, there is often tension between the client's standpoint and the counsellor's goals:

Table 9.1 Interactive issues in counselling

Client's standpoint		Counsellor's goals
Existing in the moment	vs	Active forward planning
Deep dependency needs	vs	Independence
Internalised powerlessness	vs	Response... ability
Socially learned and culturally reinforced sexual passivity	vs	Sexually assertive behaviour
Selflessness	vs	Self-protection
Primacy of needs of others and submission to the sexual desires of partners	vs	Self-regard
Importance of status and identity as mother in the community	vs	Childlessness

It should also be noted that fear of HIV as a motivating factor for change often backfires. If the anxiety level is too low then concern is not aroused and there will not be enough motivation to change. Conversely if scare and fear tactics are the main techniques used they can seem so frightening that they must be ignored or rejected. For women I have worked with, both of these extremes have appeared. They have either been overwhelmed and immobilised by the contradictions as they surface or, for many, the spectre of HIV is placed along a continuation of life-long traumas which they have had to survive, and HIV becomes just another one. By becoming desensitised and fatalistic about their lives women protect themselves against the impact and potential consequences of the virus.

The powerlessness these women often feel is a psychological phenomenon which also has social roots. Often their oppression is suffered on an economic, political and psychological level. Most of the women with whom I have worked have internalised their powerlessness which often leaves them with feelings of despair, defeatism and fatalism. It leads them to accept aspects of their world and themselves which they know to be contrary to their own best interests.

In conclusion, the work of HIV prevention is a far more challenging task than we initially imagined. Education on HIV transmission and increasing availability of condoms will have little effect on preventing heterosexual transmission if the underlying psychological dynamics are not addressed. Women can often be trapped by their sexual passivity, their perceptions of the rewards of parenthood and pregnancy, their sense of being unable to act in the world and their very low self-esteem. In this context, the modification of sexual behaviour to reduce the risk of HIV infection is a formidable undertaking. The questions surrounding women and AIDS, and consequently counselling in this area, cannot be separated from wider issues of women's role in society. To be effective in our attempts to develop preventative strategies, we must recognise and address the social, political and psychological influences on women.

REFERENCES

Dorn, N., Henderson, S. and South, N. (1991) *AIDS: Women, Drugs and Social Care*, London: Falmer Press.
Miller, J.B. (1976) *Towards a New Psychology of Women*, USA: Bantam Books.

10 Women as carers

Jane Wilson

'Women as carers' is certainly not a new phenomenon. Historically women have always been carers. In pre-capitalist periods women combined this role with a direct contribution to production. The subsequent evolving division of labour whereby women either 'cared' at home, entered the labour market in low-paid service work or were streamlined into the bottom rung of careers often associated with their caring skills (e.g. nursing, teaching, social work), is evidence not only of their ability in this arena but of the value society has placed on their contribution. At present women deliver this care both within their family systems and in society as a whole and I have little doubt that it will be women who will increasingly carry the weight of caring for those affected by HIV and AIDS.

After nearly a decade of responding to the human needs of an inhuman virus, many women, whether they are caring professionally or personally, have begun to voice concerns about how they function in this role.

The rapid progression of this epidemic is mirrored by the accelerated response to the needs of those touched by it. Many, many women have stated that the growing emotional intensity of the work and the increased pressure generated by it have stretched their coping and caring skills much further than they had anticipated.

To simply highlight and praise the excellent contribution made by women in this area would be insufficient, particularly given the questions women are raising about this issue. Nor does it seem appropriate solely to examine the particular issues generated by the virus. To understand fully the complexity of women's relationship to their caring role I have cast the net wider and drawn on material from female psychology and gender socialisation in an attempt to elicit themes which seem to underlie our current situation.

To begin with, who are the women who are caring?

a   Women living with HIV and AIDS who, via self-help groups or informal
    support networks, share their strength, experience and vision with others

affected by the virus. These women will continue to come forward regardless of whether they are unsupported or under-supported in this task.

b Women in their family and social settings who, as mothers, wives, partners, sisters, grandmothers, daughters and friends, carry the emotional and practical responsibility for tending to their loved ones with the virus. These women will continue to carry this burden whether or not sufficient back-up or respite care is available.

c Women in the community or in statutory settings who provide their caring either as low-waged support and ancillary workers or as unpaid volunteers. The value society places on women's work is often reflected in their pay packets. Along with this, the increasing trend towards using volunteers to offset the escalating cost of caring for those with the virus will mean increasing demands on women who constitute the majority of volunteers in the community. The exception to this is the commendable work done by the gay male community. They have been the vanguard in mobilising an effective response to AIDS, the introduction of the 'buddy' befriending system being one example.

d Women working in health, social services and the voluntary sector who have brought their caring skills to the fore in an effort to support those affected by HIV and to halt its spread. However, these women, in disproportionate numbers, occupy the fieldwork and coalface positions rather than the managerial or policy-forming ones.

Unequivocally, the caring provided by all these women should be acknowledged and validated. To do so would mean translating into active reality the requisite support mechanisms to sustain such work. However, most women claim that they do not experience their contributions as well supported, if supported at all (Dorn *et al.* 1991).

While it is important to comment on the limited support, recognition and validation that women as carers receive, it may be more fruitful to examine our collusion in this. This is not to say that men receive adequate support when providing caring, for clearly they do not. Nonetheless, I would suggest that the processes and dynamics involved may be quite different. It is the specific ways in which women have come to perceive their identity as women and its impact on their role as carers that I would like to explore.

The issue surely, is not women's ability to care. We do that well... it's easy. The dis . . . ease seems to surface around our ability to care equally for ourselves as well as for others in the face of an epidemic that will continue to exact a toll on our psyche, our souls, our emotions and our spirit.

Paradoxically, women involved in this work talk constantly about the need for support while at the same time feeling unable to assert these needs in a way that allows them to be met. They often comment on the ways in which they 'snooker' themselves in this regard and it may be useful to examine some 'myths' about women which may contribute to this situation.

Where better to begin than with human nature? There is a longstanding assumption that our nature is fixed by gender. In addition, declarations about exactly what is fixed and what is open to change have often not been ours to make.

I began by stating that historically women have always been carers. However, history and the social organisations which shape it do not necessarily follow laws of nature. Nonetheless, history has often been equated with nature and 'women as carers' has been viewed as a natural phenomenon rather than a social one.

Nancy Chadrow, in her book entitled *The Reproduction of Mothering* (1987), argues an eloquent case for the re-evaluation of our assumed natural abilities. She claims that our internal psychological make-up and our early social learning are shaped by our primary relationship with our mothers who, of course, are women. This foundation is structurally reproduced through the generations and solidified in our social organisation. What appears natural and fixed is in essence historically determined. We are seen to do what we do without effort or exertion. Nonetheless, caring is a psychological and social attribute of women not a biological one like childbearing.

If we assign our caring attributes to nature or natural ability there is an obvious consequence. You do not need to build in a great deal of support for something that will occur naturally. Women workers also tend to believe this, questioning themselves and their capabilities if they feel the need for support, let alone dare to ask for it.

On the subject of recognition and validation for caring, the issue of status should be explored. Few would argue that division of labour exists between men and women. On the basis of our presumed natural ability, the role of caring is overwhelmingly ascribed to women. Although it is seen as a necessary activity for the healthy functioning of society, it is often separated off from the 'mainstream' activities of men. Thus, women acting 'in' the world are often seen as a supportive element to the male task of acting 'upon' and changing the world. The assumption that caring is secondary to the primary 'productive' role reserved for men will have an impact on how we view both our work and ourselves. If women internalise a devalued sense of their role it will have a considerable impact on their self-esteem and self-worth. If we listen to women describe their work there is no doubt that they often perform their caring with an uneasy sense that what they do is not as useful as what men do. They may actually collude with denying the importance and significance of their own experience and activities.

Jean Baker Miller aptly described this phenomenon in her book *Towards a New Psychology of Women* when she states:

> To care for the ill and the disabled who are often marginalised from the mainstream, to rear children who have not yet moved into the mainstream and to service men during the hours when they are out of the mainstream so that they can go back into the mainstream can have the effect of placing caring on the periphery of what is seen as the real world productive 'doing' in the way that men 'do'.

(Miller 1976: 53)

Miller draws the conclusion that the relegation of caring to a peripheral role creates a double bind for many women, whereby women's caring activities are seen as secondary and yet women are expected to feel fully valued persons in society.

This demarcation, whereby men are perceived as 'doers' and women as givers and carers, contains within it other differences based on the way each of the sexes assesses their relationship to their role. Men can be seen to evaluate themselves on their achievements which are usually external, concrete and easily measured. Their self-image and self-worth will often be shaped by their successes. Women, however, will often tend to evaluate themselves on the quality and quantity of their caring which is less visible, less easily measured and less valued by society. If they feel that their giving is insufficient or inadequate, their self-image and self-worth will suffer.

To go deeper, this attachment of women's identity to their role as carers can produce even further difficulties. The social assumption that women's caring is ever-plentiful can leave many women feeling that others are asking too much of them. This dilemma may give rise to feelings of resentment which may in turn lead to the development of internal conflicts. Feelings of resentment about caring may easily give rise to guilt, as women often believe they should be able to fulfil this role without difficulty. In order to avoid guilt feelings they may deny that they actually resent these excess pressures. Consequently, it becomes very difficult to take even small steps to limit demands on what they can cope with. Women will then find themselves trapped in the scenario 'I can't give any more but I don't feel allowed to stop.'

If these themes of human nature, status and identity are pertinent – and I believe they are – and if we can relate to some, if not all, of the dynamics which they engender, what then are the implications to be drawn for women involved in caring for those with HIV and AIDS, particularly those women who are themselves HIV positive?

Quite simply, it could be said that women coming into this arena may find themselves encased in imperative 'shoulds', suppressed needs and conflicting priorities which will leave them much more vulnerable to burn-out and stress-related illnesses than men.

If we collude with the premise that our 'natural' ability to care will see us through, then support will continue to be either non-existent, haphazard, inferior or, as one senior manager described it, 'a luxury which could not be afforded'.

If we also collude with the assumption that our caring is worthy but less important than the productive work men do, not only will we fail to honour and recognise our own worth but we will devalue the contribution of other women as well.

If we limit the contours of our identity to our giving, we not only become unable or uncomfortable with receiving but we also disown the other significant attributes we may have.

It is not my intention to diminish the importance of our caring. I am proud of our strengths and qualities in this regard. We are resonant to the needs of others and feel strongly that those needs can and should be attended to. What I am questioning is how well we are able to demonstrate our capacity to care, while also allowing our own needs to be met and, more specifically, to legitimate our right to have such needs.

We need to give ourselves permission to take time out and recharge our batteries. We also need to support our colleagues in quality 'self-care' and if necessary confront each other when attitudes and other priorities undermine our ability to practise good 'self-care'.

In several workshops which the Women and HIV/AIDS Network have held, and in research carried out on the subject of women as carers (Institute for the Study of Drug Dependence 1989), what repeatedly seems to surface are the following demands:

a formal and public acknowledgement of the role that women play;
b clear guidelines as to what their responsiblities and tasks are in the work they undertake;
c comprehensive supervision which covers developmental, educational and supportive functions and not merely monitoring ones, and supervision which includes components which are organisational, professional and personal;
d protected time and consistent arrangements which would allow the above to happen;
e access to both formal and informal consultation in work time to both advance the direction of the work and provide particular expertise on difficulties that arise within the content of the work;
f provision of a range of support structures which would allow a measure

of individual choice so that carers can defuse and discharge the emotionally laden issues which surface;

g sufficient back-up cover to allow respite from caring so that all carers can renew and recharge their batteries;

h adequate 'time-out' to process feelings of grief and bereavement which will escalate in time as more people fall ill and die;

i provision for one-off or ongoing training at all levels to further develop knowledge, skills and competence in this rapidly shifting field;

j substantial increase in funding for the implementation of the above which would reflect a commitment to 'caring for carers' by funding bodies;

k opportunities for women to bring their experience and expertise into the decision-making arena, allowing them full participation in shaping the direction and development of services.

While these recommendations are primarily for 'professional' carers, it is also important that we acknowledge the work done by 'informal' carers and recognise the need to provide both respite and support for the large number of women who are shouldering this responsibility and will do so increasingly as the epidemic progresses.

The advent of HIV and AIDS has placed many social issues in the limelight for re-evaluation and the concerns for women as carers, along with the support needs of all workers and carers, should have a rightful place on that agenda. The re-evaluation of our status and role in society and the demand that all our human potential should be allowed to develop and be recognised can only be a constructive move forward.

To contribute fully in the struggle to halt the spread of HIV and AIDS and care for those affected by it will require us to make just such a re-evaluation. 'Doing good and feeling bad' (Miller, 1976) just isn't good enough.

REFERENCES

Chadrow, N. (1987) *The Reproduction of Mothering: Psychoanalysis and the Sociology of Gender*, USA: University of California Press.

Dorn, N., Henderson, S. and South, N. (1991) *'AIDS, Women, Drugs and Social Care'*, London: Falmer Press.

Institute for the Study of Drug Dependence (1989) *Women, HIV, Drugs and the Needs of Carers* (Unpublished research findings).

Miller, J.B. (1976) *Towards a New Psychology of Women*, USA: Beacon Books.

Part V
Feelings and needs

11 Feelings and needs of women who are HIV positive

Kate Bisset and Jennifer Gray

HIV, the virus that causes AIDS, is invisible without the aid of electron microscopy, yet it has the potential to precipitate every conceivable emotion. For some people its initial invisibility increases its sinister presence and fear-evoking potential. For others, it allows scope for denial and the familiar coping strategy that assumes that HIV 'happens to other people'.

In this chapter we shall consider the feelings and needs of those who are HIV positive, most of which are experienced by both men and women. We shall however highlight those issues that have particular implications for women.

PRE-TEST COUNSELLING

The emotional impact of HIV may begin long before testing. Many people who present at pre-test counselling clinics tell of more than a year's history of anxiety. By contrast some arrive 'the morning after' having taken a risk. Some are contemplating new relationships and a few are coerced into attending by partners. For some women the trigger to be tested may be that they are considering pregnancy; dreams of a future family life feel under threat from relationships or activities in the past or present. Frequently people present in response to some persistent physical symptom. Symptoms which would have been accepted at face value before the time of HIV/AIDS become, in some people's fears, manifestations of a seroconversion illness or of HIV disease itself. A small number of people present with high levels of anxiety, out of proportion to their risk, with obsessional thoughts or incapacitating guilt. They may be suffering from a depressive illness and HIV has merely become a focus for their symptoms. These people need to be encouraged to seek appropriate help.

Pre-test counselling should include a discussion about health and about harm reduction in terms of sexual behaviour and drug taking practices, where appropriate. It is essential to give this process sufficient time and the client must feel safe in the knowledge of absolute confidentiality. She may be discussing the most intimate areas of her life. She has made a conscious decision to come to the clinic. She has thought about the issues and is now taking another vital step in her health care, whatever her risk. She is reappraising her health, her self-respect, the value she places on herself as an individual. Women often find particular difficulty in giving themselves permission to do this and, as counsellors, we must give positive affirmation.

This is also an opportunity to explore harm reduction in some detail. Change is not easy and sometimes professionals have unrealistic expectations. Change comes from within and is part of a process which often takes time. Yet we all know that this virus does not wait, it is an opportunist itself. There is therefore realistic urgency regarding the need for behaviour change. The counsellor has to contain both her own anxieties and those of her clients in the knowledge that this behavioural change is rarely effected by directive counselling.

Since autumn 1990 AZT (Zidovudine), an anti-viral agent, has entered the equation for the individual weighing up the pros and cons of testing. In the past there was no physical treatment to prevent progression in people who were HIV positive but well. Now AZT may be offered to HIV positive individuals who have no symptoms but who already show signs of significant immune damage when their blood is tested. AZT may be prescribed in an attempt to delay or halt progression to symptomatic disease. Pentamidine or Co-trimoxazole, agents used as prophylaxis against PCP *(Pneumocystis carinii* pneumonia), may also be offered to this group. These advances give an added reason for considering having an HIV test.

During counselling it is important to consider how long ago the person was at risk. If the risk was very recent, that is within the last two years, and the person is infected, there will be very little chance of immune damage at this stage (Moss and Bacchetti 1989). Therefore, there may be less medical advantage in being tested and the decision may well lie in the balance of the emotional pros and cons. In future this may be different, as there will continue to be significant medical advances which may allow treatment at an earlier stage of the infection.

Perhaps the most difficult and also the most fundamental question facing anyone considering being tested is whether the personal resources and social support network, necessary to survive and live with a positive result, are available. The knowledge of being infected may change the whole pattern of someone's life and shatter dreams for the future. Clearly the situation is even more complex for pregnant women who have to consider an unborn child. For some, the uncertainty around their HIV status becomes overwhelming and immobilising, to the extent that the risk of a positive result, devastating as that would be, is preferable to the distress of not knowing. Some are clear they must know, while others are definite and insightful that they are not ready to be tested. These individual feelings must be respected, whilst acknowledging that they may well change in the future.

In times of stress we look to familiar coping strategies. These may include alcohol, drugs, seeking support from a partner, a friend or a professional, or joining a support group. Some coping mechanisms can be constructive, others less so. Some are positively destructive and potentially jeopardising to health. For some people, testing may be counter-productive to individual and public health if a positive result escalates drug use and precipitates a return to needle-sharing or prostitution.

Many people seem to believe that testing carries some sort of magical protection believing that as long as they keep having tests they will be alright, at the same time exposing themselves and possibly others to continuing risk. Others may believe that a negative test offers absolution in terms of returning to a partner after being unfaithful. There is clearly a wide range of attitudes and responses to testing.

People often find it difficult that they may have to wait some time before having a test. Currently the only test available is one for antibodies to the virus rather than for the virus itself and we cannot say for certain how long it may take after exposure for antibodies to show in the blood. We advise people to wait at least three months before testing for a negative result to be in any way valid. We offer testing up to a year after the last known risk so that a negative result will be as conclusive as possible. This waiting period can be an anxious and distressing time.

Pre-test counselling needs to be highly skilled and sensitive. In the midst of confronting the emotional issues surrounding the implications of being tested, people also have to absorb medical information in order to make an informed decision. Realistically all this takes time to process and clients should not feel under any pressure from the counsellor to make a decision. Women in early pregnancy are in a different situation. There is an inevitable time pressure to make a decision about testing, unless the woman is clear that she would wish to continue the pregnancy irrespective of the result. Hopefully the individual will reach an informed decision once all these questions have been explored. Great relief can be experienced when that decision is made.

For those proceeding with testing there is a week to wait for the result. Some of our clients tell us that this was the worst week of their lives. It is important to discuss coping strategies and to make available contact telephone numbers and support during this time.

POST-TEST COUNSELLING

There can be joyful moments when people receive negative results. They are often very emotional. They have confronted their possible risk, held on despite their fear and anxiety, and fortunately found themselves to be sero-negative. They literally skip out of the clinic, waving goodbye, hoping never to see us again, and set forth to lead the rest of their lives. Some are on the verge of new relationships, others starting families, and hopefully all will assume an increased awareness of health issues and self-respect.

It may well have taken a lot of courage and cancelled appointments to get as far as the clinic. This ambivalence is secondary to the fear of the opposite scenario – that of being at the receiving end of a positive result. The scene is very different for both the giver and the receiver of such a result. The result will have arrived at the counsellor's desk. There is an awful sinking feeling as the impact of that result hits home, the memory of the individual tested, the fear and dread that has been shared, which the counsellor now knows to be a reality. You await their arrival with apprehension. People returning for results report that they study your face as you come to meet them in the waiting room. How to appear neutral? Then in the privacy of the room you tell them the result. As far as HIV antibody testing is concerned, there is no in-between. It is not possible to have a 'shade' or a 'touch' of HIV. If the result is positive, there is no going back, hence the paramount importance of pre-test counselling. You can't undo the test and you can't undo the telling.

Almost the worst imaginable scenario occurs when a women has both a positive HIV antibody result and almost simultaneously a positive pregnancy test. Not only has she to process her HIV result in the light of her own mortality but somehow also to consider the implications for the unborn child. In order to be able to make an informed decision about the pregnancy, her immunological status has to be assessed (see Chapter 4). She enters the world of CD4, T4, AZT, ddI, NMR, P300, Hb, WBC, Platelets, Antibodies, Antigens, in other words – 'HIV speak'. What on earth does all this mean for herself and her baby? In a very short space of time the mother has to work through the impact of a positive result and achieve a working understanding of immunology, virology and therapeutics to name but a few. All this while she is most likely to be in a state of shock after receiving her positive result.

RESPONSES TO A POSITIVE DIAGNOSIS

We have the agreement of a number of women to tell their tale. The names are changed; their stories may be depressingly familiar. Over many months and years every emotion may be experienced by the woman who is HIV positive and coping strategies may range from initial denial to ultimate acceptance.

During the early weeks following her positive result, Isobel was unable to talk about her feelings. However, she was able to release some of the pain by writing poems. Both she and her partner heard their positive results the same week. They both attempted denial, Isobel by obsessively cleaning the house and isolating herself, her partner by returning to a chaotic lifestyle, his drug-taking escalating. They were both trying to escape from the reality of their situations. Domestic violence arose from their fear and anxiety and eventually they separated.

Earlier we referred to the shock experienced by those receiving a positive result. Some describe feeling stunned, others numbed.

Isobel wrote:[1]

> My doctor was talking to me
> but it was as if she was dumb
> I couldn't hear her, I was looking at her
> but it was as if I was staring right through her,
> she must have spoken to me for about an hour
> but I did not hear one word.
> She gave me a prescription, I got up and walked
>   out,
> I felt so very numb and scared.

Often, the next reaction is one of a desire to escape from the reality of the situation, by whatever means familiar from the past such as alcohol, valium, heroin or denial. A wish to escape from reality is often not a new feeling for many with an addiction problem. Some drug users embark on a career of addiction at a very early age, secondary to unhappiness in their home and the pervading feeling of hopelessness and helplessness about the future in terms of employment and obtaining a better quality of life. For some, taking pills was just something they wanted to try but for many it was a means of escape and a coping strategy which they have followed for many years. Perhaps, therefore, it is unrealistic to think that, when faced with this devastating news, a person will suddenly cope in a different way.

For many, denial is a familiar coping mechanism. Many have no experience of working through difficult and painful feelings and so the process of denial may continue for a long time. The client may disappear from support services with a plan to put the knowledge of their HIV positivity to the back of their minds. For some this works well, for others it is unrealistic and they suffer loneliness and isolation. Many HIV positive people say that not a day goes by when their awareness of being positive is not around. Many describe feeling as if it is all a horrible nightmare, just hoping that they are going to wake up soon.

Isolation can be within oneself or in relation to the community. One woman described feeling as if she were living behind one-way glass – she could see the world and the people outside but it felt as if nobody could see in.

Isobel also experienced hurt:

> No length of time can take the hurt away
> the hurt I feel inside
> I want to run away, just to run and hide.

Many people 'search' as a way of keeping hope alive. They will try anything – such as vitamins or trace elements – most of which are untried and untested. This may seem irrational when some are sceptical about taking AZT on the grounds of side-effects. However, they know AZT is not a cure and the untested products can still offer a glimmer of hope.

Bargaining is also attempted. A grandmother revealed that she had found herself bargaining with God – 'Do something awful to me and let my grandchild be all right', she prayed. Anger is often very much in evidence and free-floating. It may be disguised although occasionally it is identified as 'Why has this happened to me? Why me?' The anger may be vented in many directions, for example at the medical and dental professions, the DSS, the police, the media, society which has stigmatised the infection. There are often valid reasons for being angry with these agencies, where there may be considerable ignorance and fear. Although generally it seems that people understand and accept how the virus is transmitted, many are reluctant to accept the ways in which it is not transmitted. Some people may have an irrational fear of HIV and AIDS and this can include professionals.

In addition to these legitimate targets for peoples' anger, their anger is also saying 'I'm angry about dying'. This is often expressed directly at the people who are closest and dearest to the HIV positive person and sometimes at the professional. We must be strong enough to allow and facilitate expression of this anger in a way which is not destructive to health, to freedom and to relationships.

Isobel wrote about her anger:

> I want to scream aloud
> I feel so bitter, but that is not right
> My stomach churns and I feel so tight.
> The thoughts in my head are anger
> I want to take them out on everyone
> I want to hit out and fight with them

I hate these thoughts, I want them to go away
But they won't,
They want to stay
And the anger is getting worse.

Unexpressed and internalised anger may turn to depression. We have often heard women saying 'I don't feel angry, I've nobody to blame but myself.' These feelings of self-blame are often associated with low self-esteem. Many say that since they have known about having the virus they feel 'dirty'. Society has certainly colluded in allowing people to feel this way. Another woman felt isolated from her physical self and said 'My body feels like a stranger to me.'

Some have difficulty sleeping, experience loss of appetite, loss of concentration, interest and motivation. Some lose interest in sex and this is often associated with a fear of transmitting the virus. Many feel helpless, powerless and despairing.

All these feelings – shock, denial, isolation, anger and depression – are common in people suffering from loss. A positive diagnosis leads to feelings of loss of health, loss of self-esteem, loss of sexual expression, loss of any certainty about the future. For many whose health remains good, there is nothing concrete to grapple with. This interferes with working through the grief process and must make the final stage of acceptance difficult to attain.

There is a fear of facing the world after getting a positive result. Some people are convinced that others must know they have the virus just by looking at them. They are frightened of becoming ill. One woman said 'I know this sounds crazy but I'm too scared of dying to live anymore.'

Those with a history of addiction or with a current addiction are frightened they will be denied effective painkillers if they become ill. They are frightened of becoming physically dependent on others and like the emaciated people they have seen on television and, more recently, like friends and acquaintances within their own community.

There is also a fear of rejection – people find it very difficult to tell those close to them, particularly parents. Parents and friends react in a range of different ways when someone confides that they are HIV positive. Occasionally they give a blank response although inside they may feel quite differently. This can feel very rejecting. It may have taken months to build up the courage to tell this person and they will find it even more difficult to discuss the subject again. Fortunately for most people, sharing the secret can bring immense relief and they can move from a powerless and fragmented position to a more consolidated whole self from where they are able to make changes.

For some people the knowledge of a positive result can be the catalyst for change. Many people have successfully stopped injecting drugs and managed to stabilise a chaotic lifestyle. Some women have broken away from grossly unsatisfactory relationships. These decisions take great personal strength. Change is always uncomfortable and it takes little imagination to understand the courage that is required to withstand the anger and fear projected by the partner who is being left.

Elizabeth was courageous. As an adolescent, she lived, like so many of us, in a part fantasy world. These fantasies became reality when she met, and married, a successful artist in the early 1980s. This glamorous life was not sustained. Her husband began injecting drugs and over the years their lives together reflected that of many who are involved in the drug scene: problems with money, housing, break-up of family relationships, involvement with the police – and for Elizabeth and her husband, domestic violence and a deterioration in their relationship. They stopped loving each other. He served a short prison sentence and was found to be HIV positive. Elizabeth decided to be tested, and was found to be positive also. She experienced many of the emotions described and when she made contact with the clinic she had already worked through her feelings of powerlessness. It was anger which sustained her – anger for being infected by a virus for which there was no cure and anger towards her husband for having infected her. She knew that this was irrational as no-one knew of this virus in the early 1980s. She had great ambivalence towards him. This ranged from feelings of great unhappiness, responsibility towards him, and yet awareness of the countless times when decisions had been made and broken by him to seek help for drug addiction. She herself did not use drugs. Ultimately she decided to leave him in the knowledge that he had the support of a drug worker and also his family. The decision was very hard for her yet she was convinced that, to live positively with the virus, she had to give her own needs priority.

NEEDS OF HIV POSITIVE WOMEN

There are basic practical and fundamental services which should be made available for all those who are positive.

Primary medical and dental care and also regular medical evaluation and follow-up are essential. Specialist services, both voluntary and statutory, for addiction problems and access to counselling services should be available. These services need not be hospital-based and may well be better placed in the community.

Hard facts can dispel fear and help build confidence. People need to know that they can still hug and kiss their children. Everyone needs close and loving relationships, especially anyone who feels their world is falling apart.

Equally important is the provision of support networks. This is a virus which has the capacity to frighten us all. It is now generally accepted as good practice that professionals have peer support groups. If professionals need this – and they most certainly do – how much more do those who have the virus need a safe outlet to ventilate emotion, and also to find understanding and acceptance. The traditional female roles of being the carer, giver, and also of being dependent, can escalate into learned helplessness and total loss of self-esteem, if there is no-one with whom to share this burden of being positive.

There are women who have spoken to no-one of being positive. There are couples whose isolation has become dangerous to one another and who will reject any offers of support via phone calls or home visits, couples whose sexual and emotional lives are being destroyed by their desire for secrecy. People cancel medical and counselling appointments for fear of being identified with the virus if seen to be attending a specialist clinic. At work, they feel that they are on a constant knife edge of discovery, if they reveal a special interest in AIDS. There is no doubt that there is much casual and facetious talk around this subject. Fear of disclosure, for some people, appears insurmountable.

Counsellors need to be sensitive and aware of their intrusion into people's lives. Feelings about death and sexuality, which many of us can avoid confronting, may often surface. This is particularly difficult and potentially disabling for people who are positive, who are also struggling with uncertainty about their illness.

While some are paralysed by fear, uncertainty and anxiety, a few can use the situation as a catalyst to help them focus on the priorities in their lives. They discover who their real friends are. Some are able to re-establish links with their families and resolve conflicts which have smouldered for years. This is particularly the case with those who have been estranged from their families because of illicit drug use.

Open communication with family can be so important, especially for mothers. To actually find courage, confront the reality of the threat of illness and death, and make contingency plans for the care of a child or children goes far to relieve underlying anxiety. Endless thought and deliberation precede parents' decisions to tell their children of their positivity and its implications.

In Edinburgh more than 50 per cent of HIV positive drug users who have died, died as a result of their drug use, from overdoses or complications such as hepatitis or gangrene. The comfort sought from drugs can turn sour. The relatively innocent hash, smoked as a joint, can precipitate chronic bronchitis and weakened respiratory systems can be further depressed by opiates. People become patients. They may become blind, paralysed, demented, weak and helpless, attached to drips and tubes. Control over life has vanished. 'Did you hear that my friend died last week – we shared needles together – long ago.' Fear escalates. 'They're dropping like flies. How do I know when my time's come?' This came during an island of sobriety from a woman who escapes from her reality through drink and drugs. A vicious circle results as both drink and drugs have a depressant effect and paralyse her emotionally. 'I wish I'd never gone for a test that day – it was just for a laugh.'

In contrast, another woman volunteered 'I'd be dead by now if I didn't have the virus'. She had been injecting Diconal occasionally just for excitement. After the positive result she had a period of escalating drug use, following which she began to adjust to the knowledge of her sero-positivity, returned to college, completed her course and then worked abroad. Although she had experienced painful conflicts in her home situation she had succeeded in developing constructive coping strategies. She was more successful in adjusting and living with HIV. Sadly this latter situation is the rarer one. Life events have a much more profound effect on those who have had inadequate parenting, a common experience of drug users.

People need to regain a feeling of security and control. A support system, whether it be a partner, relative or friend, a counsellor or a support group is invaluable in helping the individual attempt to live positively with HIV.

To begin any of these initiatives, women need to be able to value themselves. For many women, from all walks of life, valuing self is new, strange, unfamiliar and difficult. We must validate and strengthen this concept for ourselves and for those with whom we work.

NOTE

1   Poems published by kind permission of 'Isobel'.

REFERENCE

Moss, A.R. and Bacchetti, P. (1989) 'Natural history of HIV infection', *AIDS* 3: 55–61.

12 Being positive

Kate Thomson

Positively Women is a self-help group for women with HIV infection. Its origins go back to the beginning of 1987. At that time I had recently been diagnosed HIV positive and was feeling completely isolated. After eight years or so of heavy drug use, I had been 'clean' for about three and felt like I'd really got my act together. All the court cases, probation orders, etc. were out of the way, I'd made new friends, found a job, and was doing evening classes, planning to go on to university: a whole new life – a new start – and I felt really proud of myself. I had come a long way.

At that time there was more and more talk of AIDS on the TV and in the papers and, although I thought I was probably OK, I realised that I might well have been at risk in the past through my 'using' and, I suppose, though I didn't think about it then, through unprotected sex which I was still having. When I came down with shingles I was aware that it could be a sign of HIV infection and since I was feeling pretty run down anyway, I decided to be tested. I never really believed that I would be positive; I think I just wanted confirmation that I was in the clear. So when the result came back positive I was stunned and completely unprepared. That is not to say that you can ever be totally prepared for a positive result but you can definitely be more prepared and informed than I was at that time. I was basically not counselled either before or after my test.

I felt utterly alone, not knowing anyone else who had been diagnosed, and I wanted to talk about how I was feeling. But I didn't really think that my friends would be able to understand, not having been through the same experience themselves. My relationships and friendships really suffered because of this distance that I felt had come between us. I was soon sick of hearing social workers, health advisors and doctors saying they understood – I didn't really see how they could if they had not had a positive diagnosis themselves.

I met some gay men who were positive and that was great – a real relief to be able to talk about my fears around dying, and other such things. Yet it wasn't really enough – there were still so many issues not touched upon and concerns which we did not have in common. What I really wanted was to meet other HIV positive women I could talk to about my fears about having children – or rather not having children – about sex, relationships and so on.

This, however, was not so simple as it might at first sound. Trying to locate another positive woman in the London area at that time was about as easy as attempting to find a small needle in a large haystack. No-one seemed able to give me any clues. The same advice each time was 'call the Terrence Higgins Trust.' I called many times but people there were never able to help – always saying they would write but never doing so. Eventually I found an advert placed by another positive woman saying she was trying to set up a support group and I made contact.

Walking into the room the first time we met, I experienced an incredible feeling of relief – of being able to let go for the first time since I walked out of the hospital where I had been given my result. By the time we left it was as if I had been able to shed most of the tremendous isolation I had been feeling and throw off the layers of sadness and fear I had been carrying since my diagnosis. Talking to other women, I regained hope for the future and for the first time I realised that I wasn't necessarily going to die an early death. I realised that HIV doesn't necessarily equal AIDS, and AIDS doesn't necessarily equal death. That was our first meeting.

From then on, and for the next two years, we met regularly each fortnight and gradually, as they heard about us, more and more women joined us. It became a real social network rather than just group meetings – we did loads of things outside the group times, exchanged phone numbers, and went to visit each other at home and in hospital. At the same time, lots of women got in touch from outside London, keeping in contact mainly by phone but also by coming down to London from time to time.

We had no funding so had to rely on the goodwill of other individuals and organisations for office space, for stamps and envelopes, and for photo-copying. Frontliners were usually able to help with our phone bills which were always very high and impossible to pay on Income Support, which most of us were on. Little by little the demands made on the time of those of us who were actively involved grew and we were often asked to participate in training days, conferences, etc.

One of our main problems at the time was getting the trust and acceptance of other AIDS organisations and AIDS professionals. It certainly didn't help that most of us, at the beginning, were drug users or ex-users, that none of us came from professional backgrounds, and that we had no experience of dealing with funders.

The fact that we were women also didn't help. Although from the start there have always been friends who have supported us, many others just seemed to be waiting for us to fail. They seemed to be under the impression that we were somehow poaching on their territory, that they were already doing everything that needed to be done. Significant numbers of women who eventually contacted us told us of how they had been warned not to approach us at all – that we were a bunch of chaotic, drug-using women. Apart from anything else, this tells us a lot about attitudes to drug users in the AIDS field at that time – and I am not really sure how much that has changed today. I suppose those kinds of attitudes just made us all the more determined to prove the doubters wrong.

For most of us, throughout our personal involvement with AIDS and with Positively Women, it has been anger – anger at people's attitudes, anger at the lack of appropriate or accessible services, anger at needs not being recognised or met – that has provoked our responses. If you suggested to any of us a few years ago that we would be speaking at conferences or contributing to books, we would never in a million years have believed you. I would definitely never have believed it of myself. It was only the anger at having sat through two days of 'experts' talking about things which didn't seem at all relevant to our lives as HIV positive women that made me, for the first time, get up and speak in front of an audience. Eventually I just had to say something about the reality of many people's lives, about getting food and adequate housing, about child care or the lack of it, and about the need to provide us with those things, before spending thousands and thousands of pounds on dodgy research and flying people halfway around the world Club Class to present the results of their work. They should instead be spending research money on looking into the important issues that we still know so little about – like how the virus affects women's bodies, for instance.

For many of us, becoming involved has been a way of reclaiming a degree of control over our situations, situations where all too often it seems that the power to make informed decisions over our lives has been taken away from us or disallowed. Becoming involved has been a way of coping with our diagnosis, of creating a path through the chaos and uncertainty that a positive diagnosis can bring.

Membership of Positively Women is increasingly diverse and the women come from many different backgrounds, lifestyles and cultures: grandmas, 14-year-olds, straight women, lesbians, bisexual women, famous people, not so famous people, and so on! Many of us were already very lacking in self-esteem and self-confidence, sometimes because of drug use or involvement in the sex industry, and having been told for so long that we were worthless; others because of having been subjected to physical, sexual or mental violence within or outside the home, often from a very early age. Often a positive diagnosis alone is enough to shatter how someone feels about themselves. Far too frequently, contact with services can make things worse because of the discriminatory attitudes of some professionals. Professionals often define our behaviour as antisocial, deviant or downright irresponsible, when in actuality it's merely the result of a rational response to our individual personal situation.

Sadly, many women are made to feel that they have brought HIV upon themselves, a situation obviously not helped by society's negative, discriminatory and inaccurate images of women with the virus. We always seem to be seen as junkies, sluts or deviants, irrespective of what we do, which again highlights how society has negative attitudes towards women who choose to use illegal drugs, or who are sexually active. Blaming women for being positive also neglects the realities of many women's lives – the fact that for many it is just about impossible to insist that their partners wear condoms, and impossible therefore to take responsibility for their own protection.

At Positively Women we try to emphasise the positive value of the different experiences we all bring to the groups, hopefully allowing people to talk freely without fear of being judged or put down, for either their beliefs or their actions, past or present. We encourage women to realise that, in the same way that there are no innocent victims of HIV, no-one is guilty for having been infected. People who have been involved with Positively Women for a while often find themselves counselling others in similar situations and helping them to come to terms with things, more often than not doing it better than professional counsellors with no personal experience of the issues. We found that this was what women wanted – to be able to talk to others with the virus in a situation where they could be frank and honest about the reality of their lives, whatever choices they were making, however others might view those choices.

By the beginning of 1989 we were overwhelmed by the numbers of individuals getting in touch. I was still studying at the time and one of us, who had until then been the main point of contact, had just had a baby. We couldn't cope. We realised that unless we were able to secure minimal funding we would have to give up, as there was no one person who could put in adequate time on a voluntary basis. Luckily Caroline Guinness, who we had known for some time, was able to make a full-time commitment and we got a grant from the National AIDS Trust and free office space from the Terrence Higgins Trust. That was our first real home and from then on it has all moved almost too quickly. Sometimes it is frightening, and we look around and ask ourselves 'What have we created?'

Currently we run three or four weekly support groups including a bi-monthly African women's group. We do home and hospital visits whenever possible and one-to-one peer support in person and by telephone. We have a children's fund so that we can give small grants to women with HIV who have children. We hope to have groups starting up outside London in the near future. We produce our own range of leaflets, and are in touch with women from all round the world. However, we don't think that support groups are necessarily enough. We will be organising far more social activities in the future because this is what people tell us they want to see happening – and we now have the space in which to hold them, in our new premises opened by the Princess of Wales in December 1990. We also see Positively Women as a stepping stone to other services – a lot of referrals come from other organisations and we work closely with them, referring people back to them, or on to them, for expert advice when we can't actually deal with the issues, or if we don't have the expert knowledge. Basically we are there to provide whatever the women want – it's their organisation.

Obviously all this expansion has not come without major problems. For example, funding never comes without strings attached and obligations – the need for evaluation and monitoring of our services far more closely than we ever bothered to do before. We have to learn to grow from a support group into a structure where we have paid workers and volunteers and women using the services. The whole nature of what we are doing and how we are doing it has really changed and we are very conscious that we are in danger of setting up an 'us and them' situation, which we certainly don't want to end up having.

I think it's very easy for all of us as women to fall into a caring role to try and take on too much and to do too much for other people. Those of us who are full-time workers have to really be aware of the dangers of burn-out. There are very few women who feel able to work with Positively Women, partly because many are frightened of being actively involved for fear of being identified and becoming public. They may have kids or jobs or family to protect. So we find ourselves doing very long hours and getting burned out, getting overtired, getting sick and then having to take time off work. Therefore we have to build into the work really good systems of support and we have to ensure that we are not overdoing it. It's often very frustrating – the services we are offering are never enough. The services that other people are offering are never enough. No service is ever good enough. What we have managed to achieve is just the tip of the iceberg. What other people working in the same areas have managed to achieve in the same way is just the tip of the iceberg. Services are still nowhere near meeting the need – there are still only a few places which actually consult women and ask them what they want – and fewer still which use that information to make changes. There is such a long way to go and so much to do.

Sickness at work is currently a major issue for us. As an organisation employing people with a potentially life-threatening condition, which could in the future leave them unable to work for long periods of time, we have to look at the implications for our sickness policy. When a member of staff is no longer able to do their job, how do we ensure maximum flexibility whilst maintaining a realistic view of the situation? When an individual is off sick how do we share out their tasks without overloading others? How do we support that person in the guilt they may well be experiencing because of their absence? How do those of us who are healthy deal with the feelings of guilt we often have for not being sick? At what point is it appropriate for someone to resign because of ill health? How can you tell someone that they have to leave, that as an organisation we can no longer justify their continued employment to funders? All these questions still remain unresolved and painful to confront.

Our fight as a support and self-help group for women living with the virus, for recognition, to be taken seriously and to gain respect, has much in common with the fight to get women's issues on the AIDS agenda. There is a great deal of tokenism and nice words which is not the same as real commitment.

Getting recognition on the agenda is not enough. Having our voices heard is not enough. Words are great and important and can save lives, but actions can save a hell of a lot more lives. What we need are appropriate services that women will find approachable, with input from women living with HIV throughout the process of setting up these services, resulting in services that they *will* use.

We need accurate information that is culturally sensitive. We need legal protection against discrimination for people with HIV and AIDS. We need more information through research on the effects of HIV on women's bodies, information which will enable informed choices about treatment options. We need to safeguard the rights of women with HIV to have children without being morally judged or discriminated against. We need to strive towards creating an environment where those of us with HIV or AIDS can be as open about our diagnosis as those with other medical conditions are able to be, without fear of rejection, blame or stigma, without the fear that our children's playmates will no longer be allowed to play with them, or of people putting graffiti on the sides of our houses.

We need more options on how to continue drug use or on how to come off, if that is what we choose to do. We need housing, we need food, we need enough money to live on. Why, when we are already having to live daily with the stress and uncertainty about our health that HIV entails, should we have to put up with all this added trauma? Just because HIV has been made into a moral issue, doesn't mean it should remain so. So, if we can't change the world, at least we can get angry about it – and we can use that anger in constructive ways to make changes as individuals where we can. It all adds up in the end. While we're getting angry and pissed off and sometimes depressed, we could do with each other's support. It is always good to know that there are others who feel the same way and who are doing things differently. Support isn't just about isolated support groups, but about people working in different areas with different skills but crossing over.

Women with HIV need good, informed, sympathetic doctors, social workers, drugs workers, researchers, lawyers and so on, but these professionals also need us and they need to listen to us and to value what people with HIV have to say, if they want to do their jobs effectively. We need to build up relationships of trust and partnership and co-operation. Some of this two-way process is beginning to happen in small ways. But it's still not happening fast enough and a lot of us are getting impatient. Not surprisingly, having HIV does tend to make you impatient. I suppose you never really know if you'll be hanging around waiting till it's too late. Sometimes I want to forget all about HIV. I get sick of it. I would just like to disappear somewhere where it's not mentioned. But then some small thing makes me angry again and I realise it's not going to go away by just ignoring it. If we know anything for certain about AIDS it's that. We have ignored it for long enough already and it's still here.

Working together and forming new alliances offers us the chance to look at old problems from different perspectives, to ask new questions and to find new solutions. Just as the AIDS pandemic has served to highlight many pre-existing inequalities in our societies, so through our individual and collective responses we can either challenge or perpetuate them. So whatever we're doing, whether it's planning or providing services, support or information, whether from a personal or professional perspective, it is all of our responsibility to get it right.

13 Poems[1]

Ruth Gilfillan

I

ARC and AIDS and HIV
This bloody thing is killing me

But can I ask this little question
Could it all be autosuggestion

Is this diarrhoea for real
Or was it just that Indian meal

I know I sneeze an awful lot
But is it this disease I've got

I was on pills to put weight on
Or was that just another con

They give me placebos – this I know
Cos my consultant told me so

I'm not being diplomatic
I just want to know if it's psychosomatic

II

Some people think the ARC I've got
Is similar to Noah's cot
They think it's just for animals see
They've never stopped to look at me

All they see is my disease
Have another look now please
She's a junkie, serves her right
I saw her jagging up last night

Well let me put to rest your fears
I haven't used needles for many years
So why all the nasty lies
Is that the way they get their highs

I had great problems and that's no fiction
That was the cause of my addiction
Now I'm drug free an' trying hard
Even though my life's been marred

Oh, if you could only see
What your bad treatments done to me
I hurt, I cry, I ache inside
I've even thought of suicide

But this is my life mate, it's my lot
No matter what disease I've got
I've got to keep going
I've got to keep trying

Even though the shit keeps flying
Why don't they look and see
There is no difference between them and me
I ain't no dog, no snake, no louse
And no I'm not a little mouse

And if it's my disease you're seeing
Look again I'm a HUMAN BEING

III

Here I am, a few years on
It was hard enough explaining where Daddy had gone
She knows there's something far wrong with me
How can I explain about HIV
I see the sadness, the fear in her eyes
Each time I have to be hospitalised
and I see the way she looks at me
Each time I take my AZT
'I thought these pills were to make you well,
So why are you still sick then, go on mum tell
Quick mum, here, be sick in this basin'
I can see within her tiny mind racing
'I'll help you mum, watch you don't fall'
and she treats me like a china doll
Then the moment for something, I was very scared
The question that I had not prepared
'Why do I get a jag mum, why do I get blood taken?'
The moment of truth now there can be no faken
'Well it's the doctor's special way of knowing
that inside you there's no bugs growing
Tiny bugs that can make you unwell'
I had no choice but the truth to tell
'You don't have these bugs darling, so there's no need
    to worry'
'But you have, mummy,' she says in a hurry
'Yes my lamb, in me these bugs grow'
'When you die mummy, where will I go?'
I don't know the answer to that question
Instead I made this stupid suggestion
Shall we go to the fridge and get some Ice Cream
Then we had a cuddle, and I said I'm here
I wish I could take away all her fear
her blood just now may not be infected
but by HIV she is most definitely affected
I don't fear dying anymore
Just for a special little girl who's only four.

IV

Quick put up the barricades
Here comes that thing with AIDS

That walking talking deadly germ
There's no way our respect she'll earn

Look out she might breathe on you
And you will be an outcast too

This is not fiction, this is fact
This is the way some people react

Fortunately some understand
They're not afraid to hold my hand

I pray one day there will be a cure
As my days are getting fewer

Not just for AIDS you understand
But for all the ignorance across the land

NOTE

1   Copyright Ruth Gilfillan

Name index

Subject index

For it is possible that a wise man may use the daintiest food without any sin of epicurism or gluttony, while a fool will crave for the vilest food with a most disgusting eagerness of appetite. And any sane man would prefer eating fish after the manner of our Lord, to eating lentils after the manner of Esau, or barley after the manner of oxen. For there are several beasts that feed on commoner kinds of food, but it does not follow that they are more temperate than we are. For in all matters of this kind it is not the nature of the things we use, but our reason for using them, and our manner of seeking them, that make what we do ther praiseworthy or blameable.[16]

ot the uncleanness of meat," Augustine notes in the *s,* "but the uncleanness of desire."[17]

delicately, too expensively, too greedily, too much. Is the really only an offense against the self and the body— constitute a wrong against society? In search of an we should turn from Augustine's confession (or rry Wills more accurately terms it in his recent saint) to my own.

he modern confession takes the form of the most embarrassing moment, told and retold

The essential disgust for the body that percolates up through the passage above was repeated, with variations, through the works of many of the early theologians who addressed the issue of gluttony; they would reappear, as we have already seen, in such works as "The Pardoner's Tale." John Chrysostom rather graphically identified the symptoms and signs of gluttony: "Discharge, phlegm, mucus running from the nose, hiccups, vomiting, and violent belching. . . . The increase in luxury is nothing but the increase in excrement."[14]

Too soon, too delicately, too expensively, too greedily, too much. It was gluttony's misfortune that the codifying of the virtues and vices coincided with the first flowering of the Christian monastic movement and with the simultaneous growth of the idea that the body was to be ignored, denied, despised, and even, if necessary, mortified into submission. The pleasure haters and monastery dwellers (and those whose worldview placed them squarely in both categories) naturally conspired to put gluttony on the same list as lust—two impulses that, if allowed to erupt uncontrolled, would certainly hinder the smooth operation of a very particular kind of institution. Even as the church fathers were devoting pages and hours of debate to the fine points of lust, to the delicate distinctions between sinful and pardonable ways of having sex, so the increasing hatred for human physicality naturally began to focus on eating—the other principal source of sensual pleasure.

Interestingly, the glutton never managed to inspire the same ferocity of revulsion—or for that matter, the same degree of interest—as the fornicator and the adulterer. But the saints and clerics understood that similar forces were at work, and they labored to make sure that comfort and delight should not get in the way of the austere devotions, the pure concentration that true Christians were meant to reserve for God.

According to an early biography of Francis of Assisi, the saint used ashes as a spice with which he sprinkled his food in order to destroy any hint of taste. For Augustine, the battle to subdue the urge to take delight in eating presented nowhere near the challenge of the corresponding struggle to remain chaste, and yet it posed the same problem: how to avoid the lures of enjoyment. In the tenth chapter of the *Confessions,* he begins his consideration of the sin by citing the obvious fact: that it is necessary to eat. He notes that by eating and drinking we repair our bodily decay, in a kind of daily race with Death, until inevitably Death wins, and the corruptible body is at last clothed in the raiments of the spirit that remains pure for all eternity.

Augustine speaks of food as a medicine we are required to take; but the tricky part is navigating the distance between hunger to repletion with falling, along the way, into the snare of

concupiscence. The bare minimum necessary for health Augustine remarks and as every dieter knows—often to pleasure. The saint takes pride in the fact that he is r to drink too much, so that refraining from drunk sents a far less costly victory than the triumph ove of food. He cites exemplary cases as a way between those instances in which gluttony di to other sins. Citing Noah, who after the fl eat any flesh that could possibly be eaten surviving on locusts in the wilderness, A these were obviously very different si who sold his birthright for a mess o unusual dietary preference was no the sin of the Hebrews, who, committed the ultimate evil bellies that it turned them a

"But full feeding," th creepeth upon thy servar a common enough fa tempted to eat a little that began with Ch that what truly r manner in whi further in O

"I fear Confessio

Too soon, too sin of glutton or can it also answer perhap testimony, as Ga biography of the How often account of one's until it has lost, or almost lost, its power to embarrass. My own story, as it happens, concerns gluttony. The particular occasion for sin was a social event in which I unconsciously or semiconsciously hurt others by my rather moderate (if I may say so) descent into gluttony.

The event was a poetry reading hosted by a famous artist, and to which my husband and I had been invited by a friend, who also happened to be the famous artist's former girlfriend. We arrived to find fifty people or so gathered in the top level of the artist's duplex loft, sitting on the wooden floor and waiting expectantly for the poets to begin their recitations.

Most of the poets seemed to be current or former girlfriends of the famous artist. And their poems were, more often than not, heartfelt tributes to his genius, in the studio and in bed. It was an excruciating performance that seemed to last forever, until finally someone said, "Okay everyone, let's go downstairs and have some beer and oysters." We trooped down to the artist's living quarters, where there was a huge tub full of beer and, we assumed, oysters. There was also a table on which there were three plates, each of which contained a dozen opened oysters.

Perhaps our subsequent behavior might make more sense if I explain that just a week before, we had attended a wedding at which there was an oyster bar with a seemingly unlimited supply of bivalves. As in some medieval glutton's paradise, the supply of shellfish appeared magically to replenish itself with every clam or shrimp that we ate. Perhaps our memory of this feast clouded and distorted our perception of the reality of what turned out to be an entirely different situation.

In any case, our friend, my husband, and I decided to do the right—the polite, the socially responsible—thing. We would each help ourselves to a beer, then make our way to the table, at which we would each eat our dozen or so oysters, and then leave to make room for the other guests to likewise have their fill.

Which is essentially what we did. Until we clearly heard someone say, "They've eaten *all* the oysters." We turned to see that the tub we'd assumed to be full of beer and oysters contained, in fact, only beer. Had we imagined the oysters? Or had our clear sights been dimmed by a faint haze of hostility generated by the cruelly protracted poetry reading? I have never been completely sure. Mostly what I remember is how quickly we left the party, and my sense of how we must have looked, as hurried and guilty as Adam and Eve fleeing Eden in a Renaissance painting.

While it may seem that gluttony is a personal crime that involves only the self, the introduction of a situation in which there is a limited food supply—as there is, at every moment, if we consider our planet to be such a situation—makes gluttony seem more serious: a sin against one's fellow human beings and against humanity in general. So it begins to seem more like anger and sloth—volatile, irresponsible, threatening, and at the very least unproductive. Consequently, it's hardly surprising that as Christianity became—as religions tend to—an instrument of social control as well as a spiritual discipline, when men and women began living in convents and monasteries, gluttony assumed pride of place in the hierarchy of deadly sins.

This was especially relevant for those early church fathers who were less interested in the vagaries of the individual soul than in the broader and more concrete requirements of running a social institution, especially that tricky one: a domestic confraternity in which a large group of theoretically celibate men were supposed to co-exist in peace and harmony. It comes as no surprise that the Benedictine Rule is very clear on, and meticulously detailed about, the regulations pertaining to the dinner hour:

> An hour before meal time let the weekly servers receive each a cup of drink and a piece of bread over the prescribed portion, that they may serve their brethren at the time of refection without murmuring and undue strain. On solemn feast days, however, let them abstain till after Mass.
>
> Making allowance for the infirmities of different persons, we believe that for the daily meal, both at the sixth and the ninth

hour, two kinds of cooked food are sufficient at all meals; so that he who perchance cannot eat of one, may make his meal of the other. Let two kinds of cooked food, therefore, be sufficient for all the brethren. And if there be fruit or fresh vegetables, a third may be added. Let a pound of bread be sufficient for the day, whether there be only one meal or both dinner and supper. If they are to eat supper, let a third part of the pound be reserved by the Cellarer and be given at supper.

If, however, the work hath been especially hard, it is left to the discretion and power of the Abbot to add something, if he think fit, barring above all things every excess, that a monk be not overtaken by indigestion. For nothing is so contrary to Christians as excess, as our Lord saith: "See that your hearts be not overcharged with surfeiting."[18]

To understand the importance of these strictures, you need only imagine the refectory of the monastery. The monks are waiting at the table. The brothers who work in the kitchen appear with bowls of gruel, loaves of bread, perhaps even the platters of meat; considerable evidence exists that the medieval diet was richer and more carnivorous than we tend to assume. Let us imagine that each monk has taken his share, and that there is just enough food for each one, or in any case the amount that the monastery has decided is appropriate for each one. And let us further imagine that perhaps by some miscalculation one extra portion is left over, and that one monk—perhaps the same one every evening—blithely helps himself to the remaining portion, while the others watch with . . . what? Disgust or contempt, envy or anger. So gluttony *can* be the mother of further sin, and is it any wonder that, under the circumstances, John Cassian placed it at the head of his roster of faults that must be overcome.

Cassian, a fourth-century monastic, founded holy orders for men and women near Marseilles and devised a code of conduct for their daily routine and for the operation of the monastery. His inventory of the eight principal vices would later form the basis for Gregory the Great's list of seven deadly sins. He was also the proponent of an early form of what we have come to call muscular Christianity; many of his metaphors describe the overcoming of sin as something like a formal wrestling match performed by "athletes of Christ."

"And so," he wrote, "the first conflict we must enter upon is that against gluttony" because "we cannot enter the battle of the inner man unless we have been set free from the vice of gluttony." We cannot begin to undertake the "Olympic" contests against our vices, we cannot start to wage war against our spiritual failings until we have overcome our carnal desires. "For it is impossible for a full belly to make trial of the combat of the inner man: nor is he worthy to be tried in harder battles, who can be overcome in a slight skirmish." For Cassian, too, lust is at the end of the natural progression of vices set in motion by gluttony, and he stresses the importance of bridling sensual temptation: "Do not pity the body bitterly complaining of weakness, nor fatten it up with extravagant food. . . . For if it recovers, it will rise up against you and it will wage battle against you without truce. . . . A body deprived of food is an obedient horse, and it will never throw off its rider."[19]

Another early theologian, Saint John Chrysostom, a popular preacher known for his "golden voice" and whose sermons on occasion soared to lofty heights of anti-Semitism and misogyny, was considerably less tolerant than John Cassian in his condemnation of the gluttonous impulse—a temptation he traced back to the doubting, ungrateful, manna-gobbling Jews in the wilderness. In fact, he saw Jewish gluttony as one of the principal obstacles preventing the Hebrews from converting en masse to Christianity.

> There is nothing worse, nothing more shameful, than gluttony; it makes the mind gross and the soul carnal; it blinds, and permits not to see clearly. Observe, for instance, how this is the case with the Jews; for because they were intent upon gluttony, entirely occupied with worldly things, and without any spiritual

thoughts, though Christ leads them on by ten thousand sayings, sharp and at the same time forbearing, even thus they arise not, but continue groveling below.[20]

The way Chrysostom reimagines the conversation between Christ and the Jews on the subject of whether manna came from Moses or from God makes it sound like a quibble between foodies on the true nature of bread. "'They, when they heard this, replied, 'Give us this bread to eat'; for they yet thought that it was something material, they yet expected to gratify their appetites, and so hastily ran to Him. What doth Christ. Leading them on little by little, He saith 'The bread of God is He which cometh down from heaven, and giveth life unto the world.'"[21] Elsewhere, the "golden-voiced" one attempts to scare his audience into abstinence by threatening them with the horror of being found inferior to women—young virgins who seem to have no difficulty in fasting.

By the time Saint Thomas wrote his *Summa Theologica*, gluttony had made its way up to near the top of the list of the seven deadly sins and—in its probable consequences—down to the third circle of hell. So Aquinas was moved to answer, in his rhetorical fashion, the imaginary objections of those who might have been slow to grasp the less-than-apparent connection between food and eternal damnation.

Aquinas begins by quoting the words of Jesus in response to the Pharisees who accused him of heresy because Jesus and his disciples did not wash their hands before eating—an essential aspect of Jewish dietary rules and communal tradition that Christ and his apostles willfully ignored. Presumably, this rejection of established tradition reflected the sensible intuition that—respecting or breaking food taboos and laws regarding cuisine—represented an important way of establishing a collective identity and of defining the other.

It is in this context that Jesus delivers his pronouncement: What goes into our mouths cannot defile us, but what comes out of our mouths—presumably, he means lies, evil thoughts, killings, seductions, false witness, blasphemies, and forth—certainly can. Aquinas interprets this to mean that *nothing* we put in our mouths can defile us, so gluttony—which essentially means putting everything we can grab hold of into our mouth, *too soon, too delicately, too expensively, too greedily, too much*—cannot defile us either. Aquinas points out that Jesus' distinction did indeed refer to the dietary laws; then he explains why gluttony *should* be a danger—it's not the food or the eating—what we actually consume—it's not what we put in our mouths, but the *inordinate desire* for food, a longing so powerful and thoroughly involving that it comes between us and God.

Perhaps Aquinas's notably soft line on gluttony may have had something to do with the fact that the saint was said to have had what today we might call a weight problem. Indeed he seems to have been the twelfth-century version of the nineteenth-century industrialist Diamond Jim Brady, who was said to know that he had eaten enough when his belly had swelled to span the distance that, at the start of the meal, he'd left between his stomach and the edge of the table. According to G. K. Chesterton, "His bulk made it easy to regard [Thomas Aquinas] humorously as a sort of walking wine-barrel, common in the comedies of so many nations; he joked about it himself. It may be that he, and not some irritated partisan of the Augustinian or Arabian parties, was responsible for the sublime exaggeration that a crescent was cut out of the dinner table to allow him to sit down."[22]

In any case, Aquinas repeatedly invokes this inordinate desire as he tries, like Augustine, to take necessity, real hunger, and health out of the formula that distinguishes between the human animal who needs to eat in order to live and the gluttonous sinner who lives to eat. An inordinate desire, he explains, is one that makes us depart from the path of reason, which is the regulator and guarantee of moral virtue. In any case, the novice overeater can relax, because if one overindulges through inexperience— because of a hazy or otherwise inaccurate idea of how much food is necessary—that is not gluttony. "It is a case of gluttony only when a man knowingly exceeds the measure in eating, from a desire for the pleasures of the palate."[23] And Aquinas returns to the notion that the sinfulness of gluttony lies in its ability to distract man from his final end—and from the love of, and the pure dedication to, God.

Warnings such as Aquinas's against excess and obsession were also invoked by church fathers not only in regard to the rogue monk tempted to eat more than his share but also in reference to the opposite case—that is, nuns (for they were almost always nuns) who succumbed to the equally disturbing and disruptive temptation to indulge in excessive fasting. These women, whom the historian Rudolph M. Bell has termed "holy anorexics," punished their bodies by starving themselves and indulging in all manner of inventive and frequently disgusting self-mortifications.[24] Though a number of them—Saint Catherine of Siena, Saint Clare of Assisi, Saint Veronica—were eventually canonized, in their lifetimes they troubled the ecclesiastical authorities, who cautioned them to be on guard against the sin of pride: the self-satisfaction they might derive from the pain and the heroic discomfort they managed to endure.

In sum, then, the specter of gluttony was never meant to prevent the faithful from eating. Although the pious were duly warned against the insidious ways in which concuspiscence and pleasure could masquerade as necessity, the early Christian theologians had a surprising and comparatively (that is, compared to their often extreme views on sex and the lures of lust) tolerant attitude toward the occasional overindulgence. The sin of gluttony *was* one of degree, but the degree that appeared to matter most was not so much excessive consumption as excessive appetite, desire, and attention: the fixation on food, the pleasure derived from taste; the self-inflicted pain of starvation; and, especially, the ways in which all these related fixations turned one's attention away from the more important and urgent needs of the soul and the spirit.

Too soon, too delicately, too expensively, too greedily, too much. If we use this yardstick—together with that of excessive preoccupation and *inordinate interest*—to identify the sin and the sinner, it becomes obvious that though gluttony appears to have become the least harmful of sins, it may well be the most widespread. Precisely because of our inordinate interests, our preoccupation with sampling the trendiest dishes at the costliest new restaurants, and our apparently paradoxical, obsessive horror of obesity, we have become a culture of gluttons.

CHAPTER TWO

The Wages of Sin

A little boy and his mother are on line at the supermarket behind an overweight woman.

> *"Mommy," says the little boy. "That lady is fat."*
> *"Shush," says his mother. "She'll hear you."*
> *"But mommy, she's so fat."*
> *"Be quiet, you don't want to hurt her feelings."*
> *After awhile the fat woman's beeper goes off.*
> *"Mommy, mommy," cries the little boy. "Watch out! She's backing up!"*

For many years, we've had on the wall above our dining room table a framed poster we bought in Tuscany more than a decade ago. The image is taken from the fresco cycle *The Last Judgment,* painted in the late fourteenth century by Taddeo di Bartolo on the walls of the cathedral of San Gimignano.

It's a nightmare vision of gluttons suffering in hell. Six sinners—in their former lives, big eaters—are gathered around a table covered with a white cloth. The damned, four men and two women, are naked, and all have bodies that testify to the sin responsible for the eternity they are now spending in the dining room in hell. The men have huge bellies, fleshy arms and backs; one has pendulous breasts. The women seem less obese than hefty and muscular; still, by fourteenth-century standards of female beauty, they are dauntingly Amazonian.

On the table are decanters of wine, glasses, round loaves of bread, and in the center a platter on which there is a plump, rather lonely looking, chicken. The damned stare, transfixed, at the food, their faces masks of desire, avidity, horror, and pain. Because standing in a sort of second tier, surrounding the circle of gluttons, is a small band of demons with a remarkable resemblance to Maurice Sendak's Wild Things. But this is not Sendak's "wild rumpus;" there's nothing playful about these devils. Their job is preventing the gluttons—by holding their arms and heads with their sharp talons and claws, by prodding them with bats and clubs—from getting anywhere near the food they crave. On one side of the anguished group, a horned monster grabs the arms of the man with the breasts and pins them behind his back.

On the ground, in front of the table, is the man who seems the most acutely aware of his sad fate and who appears to be taking it hardest. His body is twisted and malformed; neither his rib cage nor his genitals are where, anatomically, they should be. It's almost as if his body—flesh itself—has become a mockery of the desires that once drove him. A serpent coils around his upper torso and arms. Unable to stand the sight of the meal at which his companions are gazing with such longing, he bows his head in a posture of grief and covers his face with his hands.

On our poster, beneath the image—which, as it happens, rather closely resembles yet another depiction of sinners in hell, Fra Beato Angelico's later *The Last Judgment*—is a caption supplied by the regional tourist board of San Gimignano, *Mangiare bene a San Gimignano non e peccato*. To eat well in San Gimignano is not a sin.

But if it's not a sin in San Gimignano, where *is* it a sin? Nowhere, is the only logical answer one can possibly conclude. Surely (the poster slyly suggests) when the church talks about gluttony, it doesn't mean *Mangia bene*, eating well. Eating well, as every Italian knows, is a major reason to live, every human's birthright. Indeed, eating well is nothing less than a moral and social duty.

So why should we be surprised if Catholic Church officials (including, as we have seen, Thomas Aquinas) responded to the promptings of this sense of duty. For centuries, writers—among them, Chaucer and Rabelais—have made fun of clerics who preach against gluttony and then, the moment their sermons end, race out of the church before their sumptuous Sunday lunches have a chance to get cold. The alleged gluttonousness of priests was, for centuries, a sort of cultural given, part urban legend, part fact, part cliché, part projection—and the subject of enormous fascination and speculation.

In fact, there was a certain amount of truth in these allegations. During the Middle Ages, the clergy regularly indulged in a sort of ritualized gluttony, setting aside certain holidays—most notably the Feast of Fools, a chaotic overturning of the traditional order that took place on Innocents' Day, the 28th of December—for a blowout of food and drink that might go on for days.

> Quite apart from the feasts ordained by liturgical and ritual calendars, Western European clerics were known for their capacity to eat. According to the Roman Curia, priests in the north of Italy—in spite of the order to eat "normal amounts"—actually ate Pantagruelesque portions. As late as 1059, reminders were issued at the Lateran Synod of the apparently unfor-

gettable excesses that had taken place at a church conference in Aachen in 816.[25]

In our own era, in contemporary Rome, a popular piece of tourist advice counsels that if you happen to find yourself in the vicinity of the Vatican, around lunchtime, you should find a group of Jesuits and the Dominicans and go where they go, eat in the restaurants where they eat, order what they order. In these jokes about the eating and drinking habits of priests, cynicism about the piety of gourmands is admixed with sly admiration for men who have, in theory, abjured the temptations of the world and still know how to live pleasurably in that very same world. Surely, such men of God show us with their actions, with their very bodies, that eating well is *not* really a sin. And not just in San Gimignano.

Like Taddeo di Bartolo and Fra Angelico, Dante thought otherwise. For even as the theologians were codifying the offenses for which one could be sent to the less salutary and welcoming regions of the afterlife, visionary artists and writers were turning their imaginations loose on the subject of what sinners could expect to find there.

In the sixth canto of the *Inferno,* the gluttons are consigned to the third circle of hell, to a lower region and a more hideous fate than the lustful, whose sin resembles their own in its violation of the principles of continence and moderation. But—in the ranking contest that has determined the hierarchy of sin—the gluttons have outdone the lechers in the beastliness and the sheer animal grossness of their vices. At least the lustful have fixed their worshipful attentions on each other. What have the gluttons worshiped? Their roast chickens, their wine, their bellies.

In Dante's hell, the gluttons shiver in the eternal foul weather—cold, lashing rain, hail, and snow—that has turned the ground into a stinking bog. Watched over by Cerberus, the three-headed dog, the gluttons howl like dogs themselves, twisting and turning in search of comfort or shelter, striving to protect themselves and each other from the cruel climate to which they have been doomed for eternity. Endless physical discomfort is their punishment for having wasted their lives pursuing the pleasures of the flesh.

The hells that Dante and di Bartolo imagined for the glutton were, if such fine distinctions can be made, fractionally less unpleasant than another prevailing notion, which became popular in the Middle Ages and extended into the Renaissance. This was the idea that gluttons would be appropriately damned to an eternity of the most disgusting conceivable diet. According to the *Book of God's Providence*, a fifteenth-century manual of virtues and vices that is thought to have been read by, and to have influenced, Hieronymus Bosch, the round table around which the former gluttons gather is burning hot, warmed by the same hellfire that makes the sinners so thirsty and hungry that they beg for straw to eat, for urine to drink, for excrement to devour. But all this is merely the appetizer, the prelude to the hellish meal proper. Next on the menu come frogs, vermin, lizards. A whole array of hideous creatures constitute the dinner that demons poke and prod and torture the hesitant, newly squeamish former gluttons into consuming.

Of course, once-pious Christians knew what awaited them as a consequence of overeating, they realized how important it was to watch their diets, how carefully they had to control their appetites. As these dire warnings and forecasts from the world of the dead exerted their pessimistic influence on the world of the living, gluttony began to seem more serious and more deadly. The promise of a good meal would surely have paled, at least slightly, when those about to eat it considered the punishment options they might expect: terrible aching hunger within sight of the unreachable red wine and golden roast chicken, stuffing one's belly with rats and slimy worms, or lying naked in the wet, cold rain with no way to get inside, and the knowledge that this suffering would last forever and ever and ever. What a risk we are taking as we reach for that glazed doughnut! No wonder that thoughtful and even altruistic humans have found it increasingly important to warn their peers about the passing, transient, gluttonous pleasure that leads to eternal penance and pain.

Perhaps the hardest thing for us to understand as more or less secular citizens of the twenty-first century is that, for the people of the Middle Ages, hell was not a metaphor but a reality the pious could picture all too clearly. Those who had trouble visualizing or who suffered from limited imaginations were reminded by the decorations that adorned the doorways and chapels of their cathedrals. One such bas relief, on the main portal of the cathedral of Orvieto, depicts the punishments of the damned in hell—a theme that is repeated in the paintings in the church's interior.

Scholars have demonstrated that in the Middle Ages cyclical famines and periods of relative privation were followed by intervals during which people ate as if there were no tomorrow. Thus, much of the population behaved like gluttons for a short, happy season of the year. At the start of their feasts, the still sober, still hungry revelers would have had a brief glimpse of the road down which they were heading. Or perhaps that was part of the point of the feast, and certainly of the drunkenness involved: to briefly escape the knowledge of the hardness of life in this world and the cruelty of the life to come. Perhaps fear and guilt might even have worked as a spice, seasoning the glutton's meal with abandon and terror.

Your mama is so fat she had to be baptized in Sea World.

Your mama is so fat that when she goes out to eat, she looks at the menu and says, "okay."

Along with lust, gluttony is perhaps the most easily depicted, the most visual of the deadly sins. How much simpler it is for the painter to show the glutton at his overloaded table, surrounded by an overabundance of food, than it is to show the more interior, more purely psychological failings of the envious or the proud.

By the late Middle Ages, gluttony had become a theme on which the artist was encouraged to let his imagination run wild. As always, the fantasies of Hieronymus Bosch ran considerably wilder than those of his contemporaries or his successors.

In Bosch's painting *The Last Judgment,* the gluttons have become food, doomed by one of hell's heavy-handed ironies: the eaters are being eaten. In the background, a stew of sinners—with the upturned faces of baby birds and the rapt looks of the newly baptized—is burbling in a giant cauldron over a roaring fire. So much for the soup course! In the foreground are two demons who could pass for elderly grandmas, except the one in the black babushka has a bird's legs for arms and a giant swollen belly, and the other old dame in a wimple has a lizard's feet. The creature in the wimple holds a large sauté pan in which we can discern a man's head, his hand, and one leg up to his knee. He is gazing directly at us, and he doesn't look happy. Beside the pan are two eggs. Are we going to have an omelet? How nicely it will go with the filet of the naked man, who is lying there, trussed, his hands crossed modestly over his genitals; his demeanor is strangely placid considering he's attached to a spit with a horrifyingly convincing and lovingly rendered rotisserie feature. You can see the mechanism, exactly how it would turn. Meanwhile Babushka douses the man from a little saucier, presumably to tenderize and flavor the final product.

Brueghel's vision of gluttony is nearly as energetic but notably less sadistic than Bosch's. Except for Brueghel's rendering of *Lust,* which delivers a succession of small shocks each time you look closely enough to see what people are actually doing with their hands, their genitals, and their bodies, *Gluttony* (*Gula,* or *Throat*) is the most animate of the series of drawings (to be later used for engravings) in which he depicted the seven deadly sins. The caption across the bottom of Brueghel's design warns, "Shun drunkenness and gluttony, because excess makes man forget God and himself." Surely, the monsters of gluttony in this demonic landscape have their minds (or what's left of their minds) on all manner of things instead of their Heavenly Father.

At yet another round table are two naked women. One is draining a jug of wine while the second sprawls wantonly and shamelessly across the lap of a nearly faceless man. In the foreground, Gula herself—the personification of the gaping

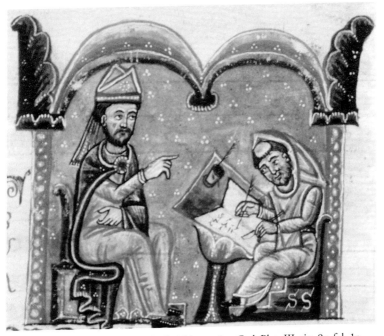

1. Saint Gregory dictating to a Scribe, Manuscript, Cod. Plut. III, sin. 9c, fol. 1r.
Biblioteca Laurenziana, Florence, Italy © Alinari, Regione Umbria, Art Resource, NY

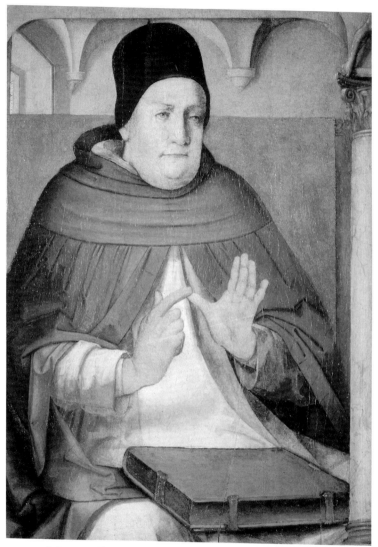

2. Joos van Ghent (c.1435–c.1480). Thomas Aquinas (1225–1274).
Louvre, Paris, France © Erich Lessing / Art Resource, NY

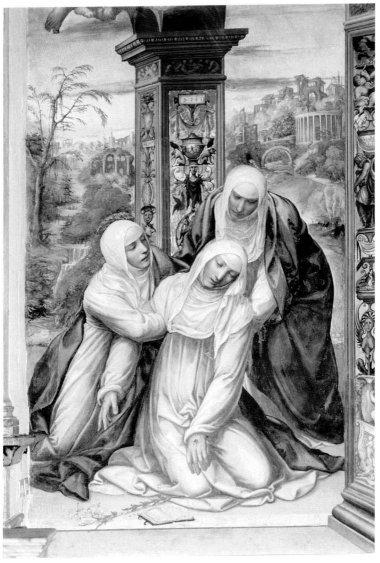

3. Sodoma (1477–1549). Scenes from the life of Saint Catherine of Siena:
the swooning of the saint.
San Domenico, Siena, Italy © Scala / Art Resource, NY

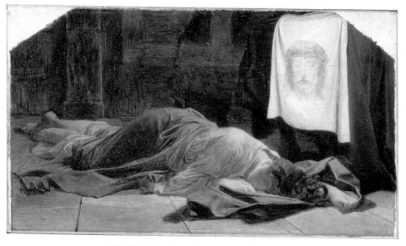

4. Paul Delaroche (1797–1856). Saint Veronica.
Louvre, Paris, France © Réunion des Musées Nationaux / Art Resource, NY

5. Sandro Botticelli (1444–1510). Saint Augustine, 1480.
Fresco. Chiesa di Ognissanti, Florence, Italy © Scala / Art Resource, NY

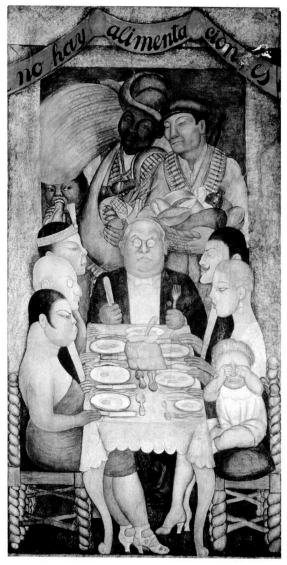

6. Diego Rivera (1866–1957). Capitalist Dinner (La cena capitalista).
Secretaría de Educación Pública, Mexico City, D.F., Mexico
© Schalkwijk / Art Resource, NY

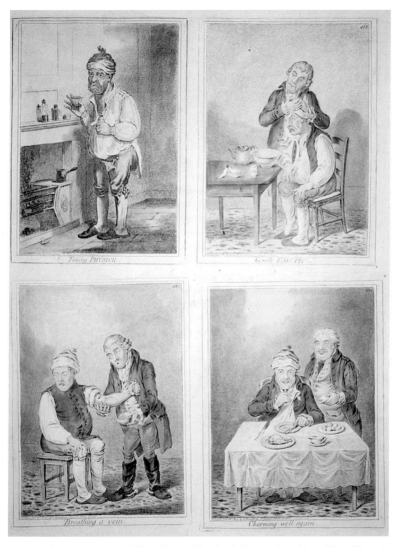

7. James Gilray (1757–1815). Taking Physic: The Gentle Emetic; Breathing a Vein; Charming well again, 1804. Private Collection © Image Select / Art Resource, NY

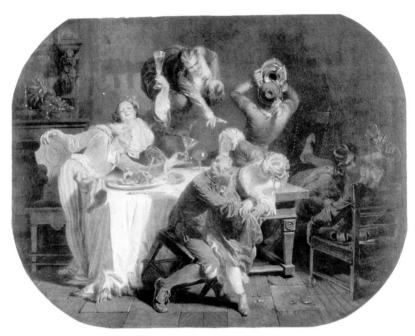

8. Mihaly Zichy (1827–1906). Before the orgy.
© Fine Art Photographic Library, London / Art Resource, NY

throat—sucks on a wine bottle like an infant at its mother's breast. One man vomits over the side of a bridge into the river below, while a demon holds his head as one would hold the head of a sick child, a tender enough picture except for the creature's beaked, hooded visage, and for the fact that the cascade of vomit is narrowly missing another man, who is swimming in the water. Men and beasts appear to belong to the same gluttonous species. Rising on two legs, a disturbingly reptilian dog grabs a cup between its jaws just as the cup tips off the edge of a plank that a porter is carrying on his back. One man has fallen backward into a keg of wine, almost everyone and everything is greedily gulping and slurping. The entire scene communicates the desperate, chaotic, overt, or barely suppressed violence of an R. Crumb cartoon, charged by a version of Crumb's unease about the frayed, thin reins of control that the mind exerts over the body.

Is this hell? Not exactly. It too closely resembles the world we know, and the disposition of power between humans and demons is not so well defined as it is in Bartolo or Bosch. In effect, the punishment is meted out by the gluttons themselves; it's not the eternity of hellfire they suffer but rather the awfulness of allowing their animal natures to triumph. What is depicted is not how the gluttons will suffer in the afterlife, but rather how unappealing they look in the here and now.

Something very similar—the sheer unesthetic unattractiveness and the social uselessness of gluttony—is what Spenser emphasizes when the seven deadly sins stage their grim and fantastic parade through the pages of *The Faerie Queene*. The passage depicting gluttony is so marvelously extreme, so exhilarating in its horror, in its desire, and in its ability to conjure up disgust that it deserves to be quoted in full:

> And by his side rode loathsome Gluttony,
> Deformed creature, on a filthie swyne;
> His belly was up-blowne with luxury,
> And eke with fatnesse swollen were his eyne,
> And like a Crane his necke was long and fyne,
> With which he swallowed up excessive feast,
> For want whereof poore people oft did pyne;
> And all the way, most like a brutish beast,
> He spued up his gorge, that all did him deteast.
>
> In green vine leaves he was right fitly clad;
> For other clothes he could not weare for heat,
> And on his head an yvie girland had,
> From under which fast trickled downe the sweat:
> Still as he rode, he somewhat still did eat,
> And in his hand did beare a bouzing can,

Oft which he supt so oft, that on his seat
His dronken corse he scarse upholden cans,
In shape and life more like a monster, than a man.

Unfit he was for any worldly thing,
And eke unhable once to stirre or go;
Not meet to be of counsell to a king,
Whose mind in meat and drinke was drowned so,
That from his friend he seldome knew his fo:
Full of diseases was his carcas blew,
And a dry dropsie through his flesh did flow:
Which by misdiet daily greater grew:
Such one was *Gluttony*, the second of that crew.[26]

This emphasis on the sheer distastefulness and nastiness of
Gluttony—rather than on its consequences for the life beyond—
is for the most part what characterizes modern depictions of the
vice. By the time James Ensor drew his version of the sin of
gluttony, the transgression had not only moved from the realm of
the dead into the world of the living but also out of the landscape
and into the private domain—in fact, to the dinner table, where
gluttony so often makes its unwelcome appearance. In Ensor's
rendition, two gross, ugly men—one fat, the other skinny and with
a long twisted nose that suggests a red cruller—sit at a table in front

of a platter on which there is a scrawny bird that seems to be, dismayingly, still alive and still possessed of most of its feathers.

The thin man slumps back in his chair, his fat friend grasps his eating utensils and leans on the table. Behind them on the wall is a painting—a painting within a painting—of a farm scene in which barnyard animals are being slaughtered. A sheep is being eviscerated, the innards and intestines yanked from its body, while a somewhat disconsolate dog stands nearby, and a pig lies on the ground, either about to suffer or just having suffered the same fate as the sheep. But what's most appalling is not the sheep guts, or the sodden, awful faces of the gluttonous revelers, but rather the fact that two diners sharing their riotous meal appear to be eating and vomiting at the same time. What's worst of all is the accuracy with which Ensor has captured a state of being. He has discovered the visual equivalent for precisely how it feels when you've eaten so much that you think you're about to be sick and still can't stop eating.

More recently the caveat that has superseded the threats of eternal hell is the threat of death itself. The idea that overeating presents a health risk is, of course, nothing new. It occurred to Renaissance writers who concerned themselves with the subjects of food and health,

> For the individual who succumbs to surfeit and riotous excess, "worshipping the belly as God," disaster awaits. For one, the

internal heat is suffocated and food begins to decay, accidentally generating its own putrescent heat. Sooty fumes build up, and the viscera swells. The fumes then fill the head, dulling our eyesight and thoughts. Then they diffuse throughout the body, causing intense weariness, and the flesh absorbs this corrupt matter. Paradoxically, the body then wastes away, having received no assimilatable nutrients. . . . With time, the corrupt matter collects in the muscles and kidneys, causing the all too familiar gout and kidney stones, of all, the sense of taste is eventually totally obscured, and gluttons search in vain for ever more delectable morsels, overstimulating their appetites, and finally eating themselves to death.[27]

For centuries, it was thought that a single eating binge could prove fatal—the Princess of Palatine (a member of the court of Louis XIV) and Henry Thrale, a close friend of the eighteenth-century writer Samuel Johnson—were among the more well known figures believed to have suffered death by overindulgence.

Now, of course, we understand that this particular road to ruin is a slower and more circuitous one, that the distance is hard to travel in a single night of dedicated eating. Yet, though we no longer fear the catastrophic effects of a single meal, the concern—and the paranoia—about the health consequences of what and how much we eat has never been so intense. We're barraged with reminders that overeating is unhealthy, that a poor diet is one of the major contributing factors to a prodigious and daunting range of ordinary, exotic, and fatal diseases. We know what our grandparents didn't know—about the horrors of cholesterol, the perils of red meat, the liver-destroying effects of wine, the artery-clogging power of the foods (bacon, butter, ice cream) that are most delicious.

Our obsession with living forever means that we are doubly affronted by the spectacle of the obese, whose flesh seems to be making a statement that the pleasures of the moment have been chosen over the promise of longevity. Doesn't that fat man want to *live?* The so-called glutton is a walking rebuke to our self-control, our self-denial, and to our shaky faith that if we watch ourselves, if we do this and don't do that, then surely death cannot touch us.

> *Did you hear the one about the fat guy who asked directions to the*
> *number six train and the conductor told him he'd probably be better*
> *off taking the number three train twice?*
> *Did you hear the one about the fat lady who wore a yellow raincoat*
> *and people kept waving their arms at her because they thought she*
> *was a taxi?*

Published in 1982, *Psychological Aspects of Obesity: A Handbook,* edited by Benjamin Wolman, Ph.D., with Stephen deBerry, Ph.D., offers an informative overview of the way in which the wages of gluttony are perceived by the helping professions. As the book makes clear, psychotherapists—and the wider scientific community—are much less likely than the general public to ascribe every case of obesity to the sorts of behaviors and indulgences traditionally associated with gluttony—greediness, laziness, and forth. The articles collected here also take into account genetic factors, socioeconomic and cultural influences, as well as the possibility that the brains of obese humans may have some biological resemblance to those of laboratory animals with hypothalmic brain lesions. In fact, in the decades since this volume was published, more and other scientific studies have concentrated on the biological and psychological nature of obesity, so that it's rare these days to pick up the science section of the newspaper or to tune in the evening news without reading or hearing about some new research into the organic, cellular, or hereditary causes and triggers of overweight.

But, as its title promises, the book's main focus is obesity's *psychological* aspects. In a series of chapters culled from essays and papers by experts in the field, the handbook considers such topics as the relation between depression and obesity, the etiology of obesity in adolescence, the problems faced by the obese in maintaining a "normal" weight, and the tendencies and attitudes—a misdirected drive for power, feelings of guilt and inferiority, distorted body image, and forth—that might predispose someone to become obese in the first place. The second half of the collection addresses itself to the efficacy of various modes of therapy: psychoanalysis, behavioral therapy, group therapy, and hypnosis.

Included are case histories in which the psyche of an obese person is probed to reveal the root causes of a problematic and uncontrollable weight gain. One man who endured a terrible childhood and who is trapped in a no less awful married life eats, it is suggested, to make himself so unhappy that his unsympathetic wife will begin to feel sorry for him and fall in love with him and be inspired to prove that she cares. In another case, an overweight woman is eating to compensate for—surprise—the inadequacies and emotional frigidity of her chilly, rejecting parents.

What goes without saying is how far we've come from the image of the devil tempting the sinner with pies and cakes, plying the glutton with the joys of the table as a substitute for—a dangerous distraction from—the more profound rewards of the spirit. For all the intensity of the medieval debate about the nature of predestination and free will, no one seems to have doubted that the glutton had a choice concerning when, what, and how much to eat—how far and how vehemently to resist the devil. At the same time, early philosophers had remarkably little interest in *why* the glutton overate—or perhaps it was merely assumed that the glutton *liked* eating.

But now that we are more likely to believe in some form of free will, we are paradoxically more willing to believe that eating or not eating is a response to something that happens outside of ourselves, something that was done to us, and that we must struggle to overcome. It's revealing of our psychotherapeutic view of humanity and of our blame-based culture that we are so persuaded that the quality and quantity of what we ingest is primarily reactive, that our eating habits are less a matter of will and agency than one of displaced response to an injury or harm we have suffered, more often than not in the distant past.

Each year, dozens of books are published to help victims of eating disorders solve the perilous riddle of their problems with food. One of the earliest was Kim Chernin's *The Obsession,* which first appeared in 1981, a pioneer exploration of the self-loathing and the paralyzing guilt and shame and terror that women in our culture so often feel for their own less than "perfect" bodies. Chernin finds a host of partial explanations for certain women's inability to get through a single day without consulting the bathroom scale. She suggests a range of causes for this widespread fixation, ranging from primal loathing of the female body that may be endemic in the species to destructive parental and familial influences, from the widespread societal and cultural emphasis on thinness to the expectations of individual men who respond with horror when their wives or girlfriends gain weight. She tracks her own familiarity with compulsive eating to a day when she was 17, living in Berlin: "I am not hungry. I had pushed away my plate moments before. But my hand is reaching and I know that I am reaching for something that has been lost. . . . Suddenly it seems to me that nothing will ever still this hunger—an immense implacable craving that I do not remember having felt before.

"Suddenly, I realize that I am putting too much butter on my breakfast roll. I am convinced that everyone is looking at me. I put down the butter knife. I break off a piece of roll and put it in my mouth. But it seems to me that I am wolfing it down." After running out of the house, still gnawing on her roll, she cut the line waiting to buy sausage at a shop, darts in front of the man in front of her, and runs down the street, eating her sausage.

"And so I ran from bakery to bakery, from street stall to street stall, buying cones of roasted chestnuts, which made me frantic because I had to peel away the skins. I bought a pound of chocolate and ate it as I ran. I never went to the same place." She gets a mesh bag in which to carry her food, and finds herself eating on park benches, trying to chew at a normal rate, as if she is having a picnic instead of satisfying a compulsion. Only much later, after succumbing to successive cycles of binging and dieting, does Chernin have a revelation:

"What I wanted from food was companionship, comfort, reassurance, a sense of warmth and well-being that was hard for me to find in my own life, even in my own home. And now that these emotions were coming to the surface, they could no longer easily be satisfied with food. I was hungering, it was true; but food apparently was not what I was hungering for."[28]

Among the writers who have followed in Chernin's path—and benefited from similar epiphanies—is Geneen Roth, whose books are enormously popular and who frequently leads well-attended workshops for people who suffer from eating disorders. In her third book, *When Food Is Love,* Roth reports on how falling in love made her confront the ways in which food functioned for her as a substitute for intimacy; she describes how, after overcoming her negative attitudes toward food, she was finally able to experience true love:

> Diets don't work because food and weight are the symptoms, not the problems. The focus on weight provides a convenient and culturally reinforced distraction from the reasons why so many people use food when they are not hungry. These reasons are more complex than—and will never be solved with—will power, counting calories, and exercise. They have to do with neglect, lack of trust, lack of love, sexual abuse, physical abuse, unexpressed rage, grief, being the object of discrimination, protection from getting hurt again. People abuse themselves with food because they don't know they deserve better. People

abuse themselves because they've been abused. . . . Because our patterns of eating were *formed* by early patterns of loving, it is necessary to understand and work with both food and love to feel satisfied with our relationship to either.[29]

Perhaps what's most striking about both of these passages, and about the books from which they're taken, is how little discussion, how little acknowledgment there is of the possibility that one might find genuine pleasure in eating, and even overeating. How different Kim Chernin's account of her consumption of chocolate is from the prose that might result if a writer like, say, M.F.K. Fisher were to address the subject of a sausage and chocolate meal.

During the Middle Ages and the Renaissance, it was a cultural given that the taste for fine food and excessive drink was a glutton's downfall. But by the end of the twentieth century, food had come to mean compensation, comfort, the hoped-for release from suffering, the whole list of interpretations that Geneen Roth suggests. To some degree, this widespread uneasiness about nourishment and consumption reflects the shifts in world demographics, and the ways in which patterns of shortage and surfeit, wealth and poverty manifest themselves and affect the citizens of rich and poor nations. One can hardly imagine a starving citizen of a third-world country facing the sorts of struggles that challenge Americans like Kim Chernin and Geneen Roth. Indeed, visitors from developing countries are often confused by the fact that in the United States the rich are more likely to be thin while the poor often tend toward overweight.

For many Americans, especially women tormented by the skeletal standards of beauty that the media purveys, food has become the enemy—but a very different sort of foe than it must have been to the medieval glutton. And nowhere, or rarely, in these books, do we find the sensuous appreciation of food, the joyous rapt attention with which a writer such as, say, Henry Miller, describes a memorable meal.

In addition to the guilt, the sense of a loss of control, and of course the reasonable health risks and concerns connected with eating disorders of all sorts, those who exceed the unforgiving norms our culture has established for the human body are subjected to semiconstant small and large doses of insult and humiliation, of casual and institutionalized prejudice and discrimination. Perhaps the most interesting chapter in *Psychological Aspects of Obesity* is an essay, written by Natalie Allon, entitled "The Stigma of Overweight in Everyday Life," which examines the ways in which the obese are made to see themselves not merely as inferior and marginalized but as deviant and wicked.

Presumably, anyone who has ever attended grade school or spent time with small children or merely watched children interact with other children will have observed the mercilessness with which the young treat their chubby classmates. Given that adolescence is not the stage at which we are at our kindest and most tolerant, we can safely assume that the life of most obese teenagers is an unenviable one. Yet thanks to the behavioral scientists' zeal for researching, documenting, and precisely quantifying what some might consider self-evident, studies proved that "children responded in very unfavorable ways to silhouettes of endomorphic children," and that "86 percent of those children who were consistent in their choices showed an aversion for chubbiness when tested with headless photographs of chubby, average, and thin children in bathing suits."[30]

What's more revealing—and even more upsetting—is the evidence concerning the obstacles and insults the obese adult is obliged to face on a more or less daily basis. The damage inflicted by the cruelty and contempt with which the overweight are routinely burlesqued in the media pales in comparison to the harm caused by the discrimination they face in the process of gaining admission to college and finding a job. Employers, it has been shown, not only tend to assume that a fat person will be less reliable, energetic, and efficient, but are reluctant to hire the overweight for positions (receptionists, etc.) in which their size might affront the delicate sensibilities of potential customers and the general public. Fat people often have difficulty in getting health insurance and in obtaining adequate medical care, for many doctors (as yet more studies have demonstrated) display an unseemly and unprofessional dismissiveness towards their over-weight patients.

In addition, the obese often find it challenging to carry out the sort of quotidian activities that most of us take for granted: buying clothes, sitting comfortably in theaters, on airplanes, trains, and buses, and even getting through turnstiles designed for the ectomorphic subway rider. Recently, Southwest Airlines passed a ruling requiring passengers over a certain weight to purchase two seats. In what is perhaps the most disturbing recent development of all, states have now begun to get tough on parents thought to be too lax about their children's diet. A three-year-old girl named Anamarie Martinez-Regino was taken from her home because her parents were unwilling or unable to persuade or force her to lose weight.

More and more often, we read articles and hear TV com-mentators advocating government intervention to protect us from the greed of a corporate culture that profits from our unhealthy attraction to sugary and fatty foods. Legal experts discuss the feasibility of mounting class action suits—on the model of the recent and ongoing litigation against so-called big tobacco companies—against fast-food restaurants, junk-food manufacturers, and advertisers who target children with ads for salty fried snacks and brightly colored candy masquerading as breakfast cereal.

What's slightly more disturbing is the notion that not only do fat people need to be monitored, controlled, and saved from their gluttonous impulses, but that we need to be saved from them—that certain forms of social control might be required to help the overweight resist temptation. Writing in the *San Francisco Chronicle,* essayist Ruth Rosen has suggested that such actions might be motivated by compassion for such innocent victims as the parents of a child whose overweight helped lead to diabetes, or the child of a parent who died from weight-related causes. Of course the bottom line is concern for our pocketbooks, for the cost—shared by the wider population—of treating those who suffer from obesity-related ailments. As a partial remedy, Rosen proposes that schools and employers might forbid the sale of junk food on campus and in offices. Finally, she suggests that, in a more glorious future, the host who serves his guests greasy potato chips and doughnuts will incur the same horrified disapproval as the smoker who lights up—and blows smoke in our faces.

Rosen is not alone in her belief that legislation may be required to regulate the social costs of overeating. A recent item on CBS worriedly considered the alarming growth in the number of overweight and obese young people—a group that now comprises 14 percent of American children. According to the news clip, overweight was soon expected to surpass cigarette smoking as the major preventable cause of death: each year, 350,000 people die of obesity-related causes. Thirteen billion dollars is spent annually on food ads directed at children, and four out of five ads are for some excessively sugary or fatty product. The problem is undeniable, but once more the projected solution gives one pause; several interviewees raised the possibility of suing the purveyors of potato chips and candy bars. How far we have come from Saint Augustine and John Cassian and Chrysostom, taking it for granted that the struggle against temptation would be waged in the glutton's heart and mind—and not, presumably, in the law courts.

You're so fat when they pierced your ears, they had to use a harpoon.
You're so fat you've got to put on lipstick with a paint roller.

In studies that have examined the causes and motives behind the stigmatization of the overweight, such prejudice has been found to derive from the widely accepted notion that fat people are at fault, responsible for their weight and appearance, that they are self-indulgent, sloppy, lazy, morally lax, lacking in the qualities of self-denial and impulse control that our society (still so heavily influenced by the legacy of Puritanism) values and rewards. In a 1978 book, *The Seven Deadly Sins: Society and Evil,* sociologist Stanford M. Lyman takes a sociocultural approach to the reasons why we are so harsh in our condemnation of the so-called glutton.

> The apparently voluntary character of food gluttony serves to point up why it is more likely to seem "criminal" than sick, an act of moral defalcation rather than medical pathology. Although gluttony is not proscribed by the criminal law, it partakes of some of the social sanctions and moral understandings that govern orientations toward those who commit crimes. . . . Gluttony is an excessive *self*-indulgence. Even in its disrespect for the body it overvalues the ego that it slavishly satisfies.[31]

Most of us would no doubt claim that we are too sensible, compassionate, and enlightened to feel prejudice against the obese. We would never tell the sorts of cruel jokes scattered throughout this chapter. But let's consider how we feel when we've taken our already cramped seat in coach class on the airplane and suddenly our seatmate appears—a man or woman whose excessive weight promises to make our journey even more uncomfortable than we'd anticipated. Perhaps, contemplating a trip of this sort, we might find ourselves inclined to support

Southwest Airline's discriminatory two-seats-per-large-passenger rule. Meanwhile, as we try not to stare at our sizable traveling companion, we might as well be the medieval monks glaring at the friar who's helped himself to an extra portion. For what's involved in both cases is our notion of one's proper share, of surfeit and shortage—not enough food in one case, not enough space in the other.

"The glutton is also noticeable as a defiler of his own body space. His appetite threatens to engulf the spaces of others as he spreads out to take more than one person's ordinary allotment of territory. If he grows too large, he may no longer fit into ordinary chairs . . . and require special arrangements in advance of his coming."[32] The glutton's "crime" is crossing boundaries that we jealously guard and that are defined by our most primitive instincts: hunger, territoriality—that is to say, survival.

So we come full circle back to the language of crime and innocence, sin and penance, guilt and punishment—a view of overweight frequently adopted and internalized by the obese themselves. "Many groups of dieters whom I studied," writes Natalie Allon, "believed that fatness was the outcome of immoral self-indulgence. Group dieters used much religious language in considering themselves bad or good dieters—words such as sinner, saint, devil, angel, guilt, transgression, confession, absolution, diet Bible—as they partook of the rituals of group dieting."[33] Nor does the association between gluttony and the language of religion exist solely in the minds of dieters, the obese, and the food-obsessed. In fact it's extremely common to speak of having overeaten as having "been bad"; rich, fattening foods are advertised as being "sinfully delicious"; and probably most of us have thought or confessed the fact that we've felt "guilty" for having eaten more than we should have.

Like the members of other Twelve-Step programs, and not unlike the medieval gluttons who must have felt inspired to repent and pray for divine assistance in resisting temptation, the members of Overeaters Anonymous employ the terminology of religion. *Lifeline,* the magazine of Overeaters Anonymous, is filled with stories of healing and recovery, first-person accounts in which God was asked to intercede, to provide a spiritual awakening, and to remove the dangerous and destructive flaws from the recovering overeater's character.

Routinely, the capacity to achieve sobriety and abstinence—which for OA members means the ability to restrict one's self to three healthy and sensible meals a day—is credited to divine mercy and love, and to the good effects of an intimate and sustaining relationship with God. In one testimonial, a woman reports that coming to her first meeting and identifying herself as a recovering compulsive eater was more difficult for her than to say that she was a shoplifter, a serial killer, or a prostitute. Only after admitting that she was powerless over food and asking for the help of a higher power was she at last able to end her unhappy career as a "grazer and a binger."

For perhaps obvious reasons, the term "gluttony" is now rarely used as a synonym for compulsive eating. Yet Stanford Lyman conflates the two to make the point that our culture's attitude toward the obese is not unlike an older society's view of the gluttonous sinner:

> Societal opposition to gluttony manifests itself in a variety of social control devices and institutional arrangements. Although rarely organized as a group, very fat individuals at times seem to form a much beset minority, objects of calculating discrimination and bitter prejudice. Stigmatized because their addiction to food is so visible in its consequences, the obese find themselves ridiculed, rejected, and repulsed by many of those who do not overindulge. Children revile them on the streets, persons of average size refuse to date, dance, or dine with them, and many businesses, government, and professional associations refuse to employ them. So great is the pressure to conform to the dictates of the slimness culture in America that occasionally an overweight person speaks out, pointing to the similarities of his condition to that of racial and national minorities.[34]

Indeed, the overweight have found a forum in which to speak out, at the meetings, conventions, and in the bimonthly newsletter sponsored by NAAFA—the National Association to Advance Fat Acceptance. A recent issue of the newsletter, available on the internet, calls for readers to write to the government to protest the National Institute of Health's ongoing studies of normal-sized children to find out if obesity might have a metabolic basis. There are directions for giving money and establishing a living trust to benefit NAAFA, reviews of relevant new books, a report on the Trunk Sale at a NAAFA gathering in San Francisco, an update on the struggle to force auto manufacturers to provide seat belts that can save the lives of passengers who weigh over 215 pounds, and an article on the problems—the fear of appearing in public in a bathing suit, the narrow ladders that often provide the only access to swimming pools—that make it more difficult for the overweight to get the exercise that they need. There is a brief discussion of how obesity should be defined, and another about the effectiveness of behavioral psychotherapy in helping patients lose weight. Finally, there are grateful letters from readers whose lives have been improved by the support and sustenance they gain from belonging to NAAFA.

Equally fervent—if somewhat less affirmative and forgiving—are the gospel tracts, also available on-line. One of the most heartfelt and persuasive is the work of a preacher identified only as George Clark:

After conducting healing campaigns and mailing out thousands of anointed handkerchiefs—since 1930—I have learned that the greatest physical cause of sickness among the people of God is coming from this lust for overindulgence in eating. . . . Tens of thousands of truly converted people are sick and are suffering with heart trouble coming from high blood pressure and other ailments which result from overeating. . . . Did you ever wonder why artists have never depicted any of Jesus' disciples as being overweight or of the fleshy type? No one could have followed Jesus very long and remained overweight. . . . If eating too much has brought on high blood pressure, heart trouble, or many of the other diseases which come from being overweight, then God requires a reduction in your eating.

Given our perhaps misguided sense of living in a secular society, it's startling to find that our relationship with food is still so commonly translated directly into the language of God and the devil, of sin and repentance. But why should we be surprised, when we are constantly being reminded that our feelings about our diet and our body can be irrational, passionate, and closer to the province of faith and superstition than that of reason and science?

The Real Wages of Sin

According to the National Institute of Diabetes and Digestive and Kidney diseases, a branch of the National Institute of Health, one-third of all Americans—or approximately 63 million—are overweight. Of these, 32 million are adult females, 26 million adult males, and 4.7 million are children and adolescents. According to a recent story on CBS, the percentage of American children who are obese is climbing at an alarming rate. Indeed, according to the CBS news item, broadcast on 20 June 2002, 14 percent of American children are overweight or obese. Every year, 350,000 deaths are attributable to poor diet and inactivity, and 70 percent of cardiovascular disease is related to excess weight. At any given time, 35 to 40 percent of American women and 20 to 24 percent of American men are dieting, and the amount they spend annually—quoted figures range from $33 to $55 billion—reflects the intensity and the cost of their efforts. The figure exceeds projections for the entire federal Education, Training, Employment, and Social Services budgets, and equals the gross national product of Ireland. According to a study of Optifast dieters, the cost per pound lost was $180.

Franchised in 27 countries, Weight Watchers International draws over a million people each week to its meetings. For the first 13 weeks of 2002, revenues rose 12 percent to $212.5 million dollars. Jenny Craig, another highly profitable weight loss company, reported revenues of $142.9 million in the last six months of 2001. For the upmarket consumer with reservations about the downscale appeal of such groups as Weight Watchers and Jenny Craig and wishing to lose weight quickly in a luxurious and more exclusive environment, the cost of a week's stay at The Golden Door, one of the oldest and most venerable health spas, near San Diego, California, is almost $6,000.

Given these statistics and considering the fortunes being made from our struggle against gluttony, we can safely assume the cultural emphasis on thinness is based on something more complex and insidious than esthetics or altruism. So it's hardly surprising that the media continues to bombard us with information about the dangers, the health risks, the psychological damage, and the social opprobrium faced by the unrepentant glutton.

On the other hand, it's probably impossible to tally the revenues earned as a consequence of our obsessive interest in food and our apparently unsatisfiable hunger: the annual incomes of fast food chains and fashionable five-star restaurants, the sales of such magazines as *Gourmet* and *Saveur*, cookbooks, kitchen equipment, and so forth.

Obviously, our culture exhibits a schizophrenic attitude toward gluttony. One minute, we're bombarded with images of food, advertisements for restaurants or the latest sweet or fatty snack, with recipes and cooking tips. A minute later, we're reminded that eating is tantamount to suicide, that indulgence and enjoyment equals social isolation and self-destruction. And someone is making money from both sides of our ambivalence about, and fascination with, food, diet, gluttony, and starvation.

In any case, it seems clear that of all the seven deadly sins, gluttony—with the exception, one assumes of greed—has become the most closely associated with large quantities of money, the most lucrative, the most profitable, the easiest to market.

More than any other living individual, Carnie Wilson—the daughter of former Beach Boy Brian Wilson and a member of the now disbanded singing group Wilson Phillips—embodies, so to speak, the ways in which our culture has come to view the glutton. No one, except perhaps for Oprah Winfrey, has had her struggles with overweight so closely followed by fans and detractors alike, and so widely publicized. What makes Wilson's case so unique is not only the degree to which her suffering has become spectacle, but the extent of her complicity in the hucksterism that has surrounded her travails.

The details of Carnie's story are available on a number of elaborate web sites that provide copious information about her painful and (or so we are led to believe) ultimately triumphant life history and, in the process, illustrate the ways in which this history is emblematic of the current view of gluttony. On one such site we learn that her childhood obesity was a response to her father's severe psychological problems. "For a little girl in desperate need of her father's attention, the distance became a chasm of confusion and pain. To ease her deep discomfort, Carnie turned to food."

Carnie was "always the heaviest person" in her class at school; at nine, she weighed 110 pounds. "Subject to the cool humiliation society visits on the obese," she was "teased unmercifully." The success of her singing group, Wilson Phillips, motivated Carnie to lose 90 pounds. But the pressures of a musical career caused her to resume overeating. "She wanted sugar. She wanted Hostess Cupcakes. She wanted Twinkies." Believing her weight gain had contributed to the eventual failure of Wilson Phillips, Carnie continued to binge, until she weighed 300 pounds.

By now, having so thoroughly violated the standards of the beauty culture, Carnie was embraced by the death culture and became an icon of disease, of the illnesses and disabilities that can befall the "morbidly obese" glutton. Her cholesterol level and her blood pressure rose; she experienced joint pain and shortness of breath. Realizing that she "was carrying a death sentence around on my back," she sought the help of Dr. Jonathan Sackier, who recognized at once that "she was invariably headed for heart disease, high blood pressure and coronary artery disease, diabetes, joint degeneration . . . skin problems and certain kinds of tumors. She was a walking time bomb with the clock ticking."

So, in August 1999, in San Diego, Carnie underwent laparoscopic gastric bypass surgery, an operation that was viewed live and in real time by 250,000 people. Since then, with the help and support of the weight-loss products marketed under the brand name of Changes, Carnie has remained thin—a success story that includes marriage in a wedding dress that had to be altered because she was still continuing to lose weight until the day of the ceremony. Her advice to those who wish to follow her example is: "Pay attention to what you *really* want. You have the power to change it" and to seek the help of The No Will Power Weight Loss Trio, a line of formulas including Thermo-Lift,

Changes NOW, and Power Nutrients Plus—all available for order on the internet.

Carnie Wilson's sad (or, in an alternate reading, triumphant) story illustrates the ways in which our culture has taken the difficulty of modifying our appetites and of coping with the demands of the body and transformed these private challenges into occasions for the public displays of self-recrimination and guilt, of sin, confession, and repentance—and into opportunities for earning and amassing prodigious sums of money.

C H A P T E R   F O U R

Great Moments
in Gluttony

In her brilliant and beautifully written book, *An Alphabet for Gourmets*, M.F.K. Fisher explores the joys of overeating in a chapter entitled "G is for Gluttony":

> It is a curious fact that no man likes to call himself a glutton, and yet each of us has in him a trace of gluttony, potential or actual. I cannot believe that there exists a single coherent human being who will not confess, at least to himself, that once or twice he has stuffed himself to the bursting point, on anything from quail financiere to flapjacks, for no other reason than the

beastlike satisfaction of his belly. In fact I pity anyone who has not permitted himself this sensual experience, if only to determine what his private limitations are, and where, for himself alone, gourmandism ends and gluttony begins.[35]

Fisher goes on to offer a characteristically idiosyncratic defense of one of the great heroes of gluttony, Diamond Jim Brady, a railroad magnate of the Gilded Age, who—or so the story goes—would begin his meal by sitting six inches from the table and would quit only when his stomach rubbed uncomfortably against the edge. To that effect, he might consume, at a single dinner, dozens of oysters, some crabs, turtle soup, two ducks, several lobsters, a steak, rabbit, and just to keep healthy, various kinds of vegetables. For dessert he might eat an array of pastries and an entire box of chocolates.

Brady, claims Fisher, was not gluttonous, but rather gargantuan and "monstrous, in that his stomach was about six times normal size." He was, she notes, a member of a nearly extinct breed—big men, big eaters whose appetites mirrored their social and economic ambitions. She recalls with nostalgic affection her days as a schoolgirl, when she hoarded chocolate bars and ate seven or eight at once, together with a box of soda crackers, in a state of sheer "orgiastic pleasure."

Lately, she admits, her capacities for gluttony have diminished. Though she may accidentally overeat, she lacks the feverish appetite

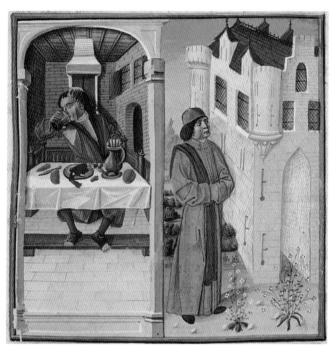

9. 15th century CE. Gluttony and Abstinence; Le Livres des bonnes moeurs
by Jacques le Grant. Fol. 11. French, 15th c.
Musée Condé, Chantilly, France © Giraudon / Art Resource, NY

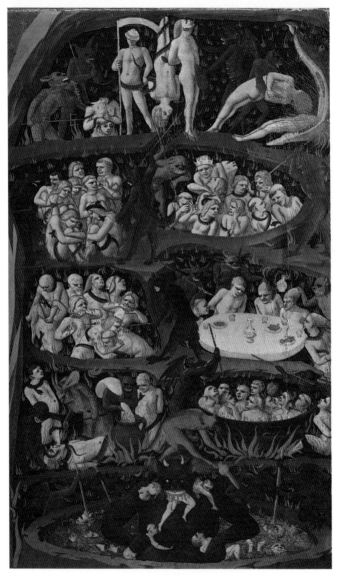

10. Fra Angelico (1387–1455). Detail of the damned in Hell,
from "The Last Judgment."
Museo di San Marco, Florence, Italy © Erich Lessing / Art Resource, NY

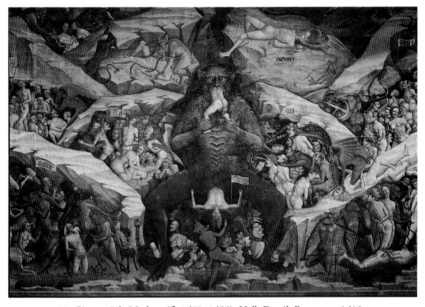

11. Giovanni da Modena (fl. 1409–1455). Hell. Detail. Fresco, ca. 1410.
San Petronio, Bologna, Italy © Scala / Art Resource, NY

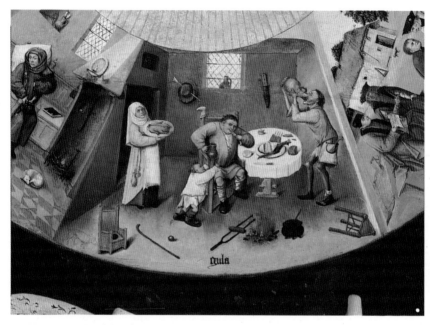

12. Hieronymus Bosch (c. 1450–1516). Gluttony. Detail of "The Table of the Seven Deadly Sins."
Museo del Prado, Madrid, Spain © Erich Lessing / Art Resource, NY

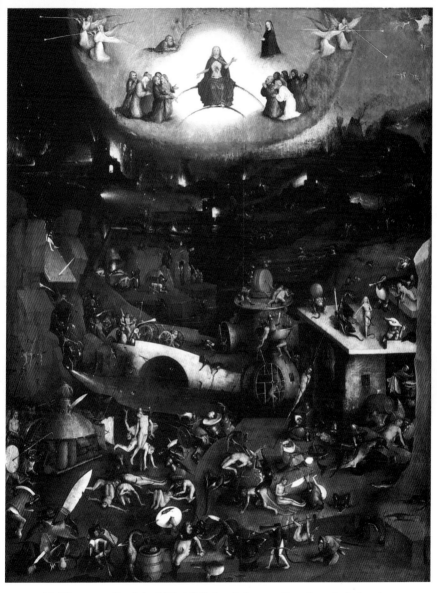

13. Hieronymus Bosch (c. 1450–1516). Last Judgment. Central panel of triptych.
Akademie der Bildenden Künste, Vienna, Austria © Erich Lessing / Art Resource, NY

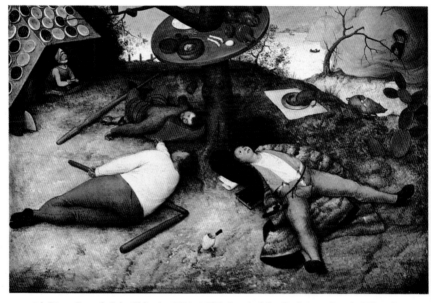

14. Pieter Brueghel the Elder (c. 1525–1569). Land of the Cockaigne (Land of Plenty).
Alte Pinakothek, Munich, Germany © Scala / Art Resource, NY

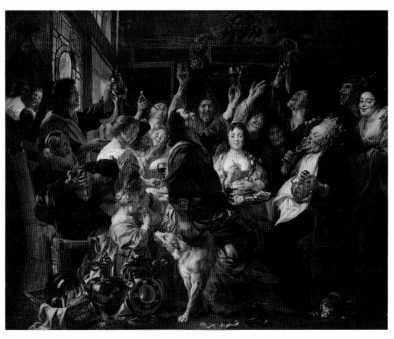

15. Jacob Jordaens (1593–1678). The Banquet of the Bean King, ca. 1655.
Musée d'Orsay, Paris, France © Erich Lessing / Art Resource, NY

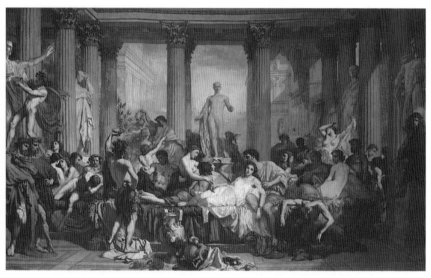

16. Thomas Couture (1815–1879). The decadence of the Romans, 1847.
Musée d'Orsay, Paris, France © Erich Lessing / Art Resource, NY

of youth, a regrettable development she regards as symptomatic of her "dwindling powers." All that remains is an enduring weakness for a brief, gluttonous encounter with a great bottle of wine.

"As often as possible, when a really beautiful bottle is before me, I drink all I can of it, even when I know I have had more than I want physically. That is gluttonous. But I think to myself, when again will I have this taste upon my tongue. Where else in the world is there just such wine as this, with just this bouquet, at just this heat, in just this crystal cup. And when again will I be alive to it as I am this very minute, sitting here on a green hillside above the sea, or here in this dim, murmuring, richly odorous restaurant."[36] This always subversive and fresh writer alters our view of this deadly sin as a fast ticket to ill health or hell, and obliges us to acknowledge it as an affirmation of pleasure and of passion.

Though no one else has expressed it quite so plainly and eloquently, M. F. K. Fisher is certainly not alone in her view of gluttony—a perspective that goes somewhat beyond tolerance and acceptance to border on affection and admiration. This brings up perhaps the final contradiction in our attitude toward this deadly sin, an aspect it also shares in common (and alone) with lust. For unlike pride, envy, wrath—sins we can wholeheartedly condemn, sins that are hard to love—there's something about the serious glutton (or in any case, *some* serious gluttons) that inspires a certain respect for the life force—the appetite—

asserting itself in all that prodigious feasting. It's not unlike our secret feelings about various Don Juans and Casanovas; even as we understand the compulsive quality of their behavior and destructive effects it has on their hapless lovers, we can't help feeling a grudging regard for so much sheer sexual energy.

Traditionally, the subject of gluttony has served as an occasion to enumerate and celebrate the quantity and the deliciousness of the foods the glutton consumes. Many years ago, while waiting for a train, I sat beside two large, appealing women who were deeply engaged in a lively discussion of the difficulties of dieting—a conversation that was, I soon realized, a pretext to longingly and loving describe the pleasures of the fattening delights they felt compelled to avoid.

"I'm always doing fine," one of the women said, "until my niece comes over with a platter of that really crispy fried chicken. That salty skin is so hard to resist—"

"I can deal with that," said her friend. "It's my neighbor's devil's food cake. She uses a pound of butter in the icing alone." And so it went.

The women's conversation has countless literary anteced-ents. On the surface, as we have seen, the *Satyricon* is a satire about vulgarity, excess, and corruption. Beneath, like so many satires, it is a celebration—in this case of excess, food and wine, romantic intrigue, and sex. Most of it takes place at Trimalchio's feast, which—as it happens—was F. Scott Fitzgerald's working title for what would turn out to be *The Great Gatsby*. The connection, presumably, had to do with expensive party giving as a vehicle for, and a sign of, crossing social class borders. But the differences between the two books, particularly in their visions of enjoyment—big houses, drinking, social status, painful love affairs in Fitzgerald as opposed to gluttonous feasting and drinking, and theatrical homosexual romance in Petronius— make you glad Fitzgerald chose the title he did. Whatever lodges in your mind from your reading of *The Great Gatsby,* it has—it would be safe to say—little to do with eating.

But the food *is* what you remember about the party scene in *Satyricon.* Trimalchio's feast goes on and on and includes dancing, music, poetry; philosophical, literary, and metaphysical discussions; an extended reading from the records of Trimalchio's estate, a display of his household goods and gods—gods named Fat Profit, Good Luck, and Much Income. At one point, Trimalchio exhorts his guests to move their bowels if they wish to, presumably so they may be comfortable and ingest even more.

Ultimately, it's the menu that readers recall, and the approach to eating that defiantly raises every one of the red flags—*too soon, too delicately, too expensively, too greedily, too much*—that, for Gregory the Great, served as indicators of gluttony's wicked presence. Even before the "astrological course"—the array of delicacies (an African fig for Leo, two mullets for Pisces) chosen to represent each sign of the zodiac—the guests are treated to hors d'oeuvres served on a platter on which a wooden hen is sitting on a straw nest that is found to be full of pea hen's eggs. The guests are each handed spoons to crack open their eggs, which turn out to be made of rich pastry. The narrator—new to Trimalchio's sense of style—is about to throw his away when a warning from another guest inspires him to look more closely and he finds inside the egg a "fine fat oriole, nicely seasoned with pepper."

So it goes, in course after course, each more ingenious and over the top than the last. On another tray are "fat capons and sowbellies and a hare tricked out with wings to look like a little Pegasus, the corners of the tray stood four little gravy boats, all shaped like the satyr Marsyas, with phalluses for spouts and a spicy hot gravy dripping down over several large fish swimming about in the lagoon of the tray."[37]

In the Middle Ages and the Renaissance, even as artists like Bosch and Bartolo were depicting the gluttons' corner of hell, writers were transmuting popular legends into works such as the Cockaigne texts, verse and prose descriptions of the mythical Land of Cockaigne, a glutton's paradise where house walls are made of sausages, doors and windows of salmon, where the tabletops are pancakes, the roof rafters constructed of grilled eels.

The animals want nothing more from life than to be consumed in the most delicious dishes. The geese obligingly roast themselves, meat and fish prepare their own flesh for lunch, and rivers of wine and beer flow freely.

The paradisical landscape is reminiscent of the land of Bengodi, which Bocaccio refers to in one of the tales in *The Decameron.* There, the vines are tied with sausages, a goose and gosling can be bought for a farthing, a river of white wine flows beside a mountain of Parmesan cheese inhabited by people who do nothing all day but make macaroni and ravioli and live according to a guiding principle something like: the faster you eat the more you get.

Among the most famous celebrations of gluttony appear in the works of Rabelais, whose farcical descriptions of the daily regimens of Gargantua and his family are not unlike popular fantasies of the Land of Cockaigne. So, we learn, Gargantua's father

> Grandgousier was a fine tippler and a good friend, as fond of draining his glass as any man walking the earth, cheerfully tossing down salted tidbits to keep up his thirst. Which is why he usually kept a good supply of Mainz and Bayonne hams, plenty of smoked beef tongues, lots of whatever chitterlings were in season and beef pickled in mustard, reinforced by a special caviar from Provence, a good stock of sausages, not the ones

from Bologna (because he was afraid of the poisons Italians often use for seasoning), but those from Bigorre and Longaulnay (near Saint-Malo), from Brenne and Rouergue.[38]

Born after his mother Gargamelle ingests so much tripe that it sends her into labor, Gargantua carries on the family tradition. He

sat down to table, and . . . began his meal with several dozen hams, smoked beef tongues, caviar, fried tripe, and assorted other appetizers. Meanwhile, four of his servants began to toss into his mouth, one after the other—but never stopping— shovelfuls of mustard, after which he drank an incredibly long draft of white wine, to make things easier for his kidneys. And then, eating whatever happened to be in season and he happened to like, he stopped only when his belly began to hang down. His drinking was totally unregulated, without any limits or decorum. As he said, the time to restrict your drinking was only when the cork soles of your slippers absorb enough so they swell half a foot thick.[39]

Though the effects of poverty are (or certainly were) among the most common literary subjects, and though many writers are (or at least were) familiar with the experience of running out of money and food, there are surprisingly few descriptions in literature of the effects of malnutrition and self-starvation. Of course, there's Knut Hamsun's novel, *Hunger*, and Kafka's story, "The Hunger Artist." But food, as it turns out, is far more likely to snag the writer's attention than is privation, and literature abounds in works that confirm the church father's worst fears about the degree to which overindulgence can fray and weaken the moral fiber.

The dinner scene that everyone remembers from Fielding's *Tom Jones* is in actuality a scene from the Tony Richardson film. In the book, Tom and Mrs. Waters do share a meal that functions as a prelude to a seduction. But it is not the seduction itself, as it is on film, and indeed Fielding makes the point that eating can function as a sort of anti-aphrodisiac, not only because it is so difficult to make love and eat at the same time, but because the pleasures of eating can distract one from romance. So the "insinuating air" of Mrs. Waters's sigh is "driven from (Tom's) ears by the coarse bubbling of some bottled ale, which at that time he was pouring forth . . . for as love frequently preserves us from the attacks of hunger, so hunger may possibly, in some cases, defend us against love." So it is not until dinner is over, until "the cloth was removed," that Mrs. Waters resumes her amorous and eventually successful assaults of Tom's shaky resolve to be faithful to his true love, Sophia.

With characteristic sly wit and grace, Fielding takes us through a sort of crash course in the history of gluttony—and a defense of hearty eating—on his way to explaining why Tom fails, at least temporarily, to respond to Mrs. Waters's advances:

> Heroes, notwithstanding any idea which, by means of flatterers, they may entertain of themselves, or the world may conceive of them, have certainly more of mortal than divine about them. However elevated their minds might be, their bodies at least (which is much the major part of most) are liable to the worst infirmities, and subject to the vilest offices of human nature. Among these latter, the act of eating, which hath by several wise men been considered as extremely mean and derogatory from the philosophic dignity, must be in some measure performed by the greatest prince, hero, or philosopher upon earth; nay, sometimes Nature hath been so frolicsome as to exact of these dignified characters a much more exorbitant share of this office than she hath obliged those of the lowest orders to perform.
>
> To say the truth, as no known inhabitant of this globe is really more than man, so none need be ashamed of submitting to what the necessities of man demand; but when those great personages I have just mentioned condescend to aim at confining such low offices to themselves—as when, by hoarding or destroying, they seem desirous to prevent others from eating—then they surely become very low and despicable.

Now, after this short preface, we think it no disparagement to our hero to mention the immoderate ardour with which he laid about him at this season. Indeed, it may be doubted whether Ulysses, who by the way seems to have had the best stomach of all the heroes in that eating poem of the Odyssey, ever made a better meal. Three pounds at least of that flesh which formerly had contributed to the composition of an ox was now honoured with becoming part of the individual Mr. Jones.

This particular we thought ourselves obliged to mention, as it may account for our hero's temporary neglect of his companion, who eat but very little, and was indeed employed in considerations of a very different nature, which passed unobserved by Jones, till he had entirely satisfied that appetite which a fast of twenty-four hours had procured him; but his dinner was no sooner ended than his attention to other matters revived; with these matters, therefore, we shall now proceed to acquaint the reader.[40]

Wry, sophisticated, exulting in its freedom to reexamine and redefine conventional morality, Fielding's defense of gluttony encapsulates much of what has been said on the subject, before and after Fielding's own lifetime, from Augustine and Aquinas through Chaucer and up to M.F.K. Fisher. At the same time, it seems as characteristic of the era in which it was written as the prose on the web site describing Carnie Wilson's ordeal seems typical of our own. Over the centuries, our notions of gluttony have evolved along with our ideas about food and the body, about society and the individual, about salvation and damnation, health and illness, life and death. However one praises or condemns this problematic and eternally seductive deadly sin, one thing seems clear: the broad, shiny face of the glutton has been—and continues to be—the mirror in which we see ourselves, our hopes and fears, our darkest dreams and deepest desires.

Notes

1. Saint Thaumaturgus Gregory, *Fathers of the Church: Life and Works*, trans. Michael Slusser, vol. 98. (Washington, D.C.: Catholic University of America Press, 1998).

2. Teresa M. Shaw, *The Burden of the Flesh: Fasting and Sexuality in Early Christianity* (Minneapolis: Fortress Press, 1998).

3. Ibid.

4. Saint Thomas Aquinas, *Summa Theologiae: A Concise Translation*, ed. Timothy McDermott (Allen Tex.: Christian Classics, 1991).

5. Geoffrey Chaucer, *The Works of Geoffrey Chaucer*, ed. F. N. Robinson (Boston: Houghton Mifflin, 1957), 150.

6. Ibid.

7. Ibid.

8. Ibid.

9. Ibid., 151.

10. William Langland, *The Vision of Piers Plowman* (Boston: Tuttle Publishing, 1995).

11. Herman Pleij, *Dreaming of Cockaigne*, trans. Diane Webb (New York: Columbia University Press, 2001), 372.

12. Aristotle, *The Nicomachean Ethics*, trans. David Ross (New York: Oxford University Press, 1998), 29.

13. Alexander Roberts and James Donaldson, eds., *The Ante-Nicene Christian Library: Translation of the Fathers Down to A.D. 325*, trans. Rev. S. Thelwall, vol. xviii. (Edinburgh: T&T Clark, 1866-72), 123–153.

14. Shaw, *Burden of the Flesh*, 133.

15. Saint Augustine, *The Confessions of Saint Augustine*, trans. Edward B. Pusey (New York: The Modern Library, 1949), 225.

16. Saint Augustine, *On Christian Doctrine*, trans. D. W. Robertson (New York: Liberal Arts Press, 1958).

17. Saint Augustine, *Confessions of Saint Augustine*, 226.

18. Saint Benedict, *The London Benedictine Rule* (Munich: Selbstverlag der Bayer, Benediktinerakademie, 1936).

19. Shaw, *Burden of the Flesh*, 75.

20. Saint Chrysostom and Phillip Schaff, *Saint Chrysostom: Homilies on the Gospel of St. John and the Epistle to the Hebrews (Nicene and Post-Nicene Fathers Series 1)* (Grand Rapids: William B. Eerdmans Publishing Co., 1984).

21. Ibid.

22. G. K. Chesterton, *Saint Thomas Aquinas* (New York: Image Books, 2001), 97.

23. Ibid.

24. Rudolph M. Bell, *Holy Anorexia* (Chicago: University of Chicago Press, 1985).

25. Pleij, *Dreaming of Cockaigne*, 133.

26. Edmund Spenser, *The Faerie Queene* (New York: E. P. Dutton & Company, 1964), 58.

27. Ken Albala, *Eating Right into the Renaissance* (Berkeley: University of California Press, 2002), 105.

28. Kim Chernin, *The Obsession* (New York: Harper Perennial, 1981), 4.

29. Geneen Roth, *When Food Is Love: Exploring the Relationship Between Eating and Intimacy* (New York: Plume, 1991), 4.

30. Benjamin Wolman, ed., *Psychological Aspects of Obesity: A Handbook* (New York: Van Nostrand Reinhold, 1982), 146.

31. Stanford M. Lyman, *The Seven Deadly Sins: Society and Evil* (New York: St. Martin's Press, 1978), 220.

32. Ibid., 223.

33. Wolman, *Aspects of Obesity,* 148.

34. Lyman, *Seven Deadly Sins,* 218.

35. M. F. K. Fisher, *The Art of Eating* (New York: Vintage, 1976), 613.

36. Ibid., 615.

37. Petronius, *The Satyricon,* trans. William Arrowsmith (New York: Meridian, 1994), 45.

38. François Rabelais, *Gargantua and Pantagruel,* trans. Burton Raffel (New York: W. W. Norton & Company, 1991), 14.

39. Ibid., 51.

40. Henry Fielding, *Tom Jones* (New York: The Modern Library, 1994), 419–20.

Bibliography

Albala, Ken. *Eating Right in the Renaissance.* Berkeley: University of California Press, 2002.

Augustine, Saint. *The Confessions of Saint Augustine*, trans. Edward B. Pusey, D. D. New York: The Modern Library, 1949.

Bell, Rudoph M. *Holy Anorexia.* Chicago: University of Chicago Press, 1985.

Chaucer, Geoffrey. *The Works of Geoffrey Chaucer*, ed. F. N. Robinson. Boston: Houghton Mifflin, 1957.

Chernin, Kim. *The Obsession.* New York: Harper Perennial, 1981.

Chesterton, G. K. *Saint Thomas Aquinas.* New York: Image Books, Doubleday, 2001.

Fielding, Henry. *Tom Jones.* New York: The Modern Library, 1994.

Fisher, M. F. K. *The Art of Eating.* New York: Vintage, 1976.

Lyman, Stanford M. *The Seven Deadly Sins: Society and Evil.* New York: St. Martin's Press, 1978.

Petronius. *The Satyricon*, trans. William Arrowsmith. New York: Meridian, 1994.

Pleij, Herman. *Dreaming of Cockaigne*, trans. Diane Webb. New York: Columbia University Press, 2001.

Rabelais, François. *Gargantua and Pantagruel*, trans. Burton Raffel. New York: W. W. Norton, 1991.

Roth, Geneen. *When Food Is Love*. New York: Plume, 1991.

Schwartz, Hillel. *Never Satisfied: A Cultural History of Fantasies and Fat*. New York: The Free Press, 1986.

Shaw, Teresa M. *The Burden of the Flesh: Fasting and Sexuality in Early Christianity*. Minneapolis: Fortress Press, 1998.

Spenser, Edmund. *The Faerie Queene*. New York: E. P. Dutton & Company, 1964.

Wolman, Benjamin, ed., with Stephen DeBerry, editorial associate. *Psychological Aspects of Obesity: A Handbook*. New York: Van Nostrand Reinhold, 1982.

Index